The aging process
needs the forgetting
to prepare us
to leave the familiar.

~ Candice James

(excerpt from "The Forgetting" pg. 80)

Also, by Candice James

Call of the Crow (Silver Bow Publishing 2021)
Path of Loneliness (Inanna Publications 2020)
Rithimus Aeternam (Silver Bow Publishing 2019)
The 13th Cusp (Silver Bow Publishing 2018)
The Water Poems (Ekstasis Editions 2017)
Colours of India (Xpress Publications 2016)
City of Dreams (Silver Bow Publishing 2016)
Merging Dimensions (Ekstasis Editions 2015)
Short Shots (Silver Bow Publishing 2015)
Purple Haze (Libros Libertad 2014)
A Silence of Echoes (Silver Bow Publishing 2014)
Shorelines (Silver Bow Publishing 2013)
Ekphrasticism (Silver Bow Publishing 2013)
Midnight Embers (Libros Libertad 2012)
Bridges and Clouds (Silver Bow Publishing 2011)
Inner Heart – a Journey (Silver Bow Publishing 2010)
A Split in the Water (Fiddlehead Poetry Books 1979)

Behind
The One-Way
Mirror

Candice James

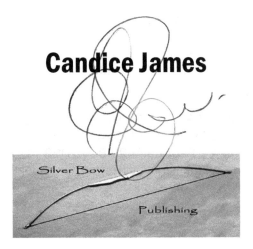

Box 5 – 720 – 6th Street,
New Westminster, BC
V3C 3C5   CANADA

Title: Behind the One-Way Mirror
Author: Candice James
Cover Painting: "A Pastoral Dream" Candice James
Layout/Design: Candice James

ISBN: 9781774030585
ISBN: 9781774030592
© 2022 Silver Bow Publishing

Library and Archives Canada Cataloguing in Publication

Title: Behind the one-way mirror / Candice James.
Names: James, Candice, 1948- author.
Description: Poems.
Identifiers: Canadiana (print) 20220428867 | Canadiana (ebook) 20220428891 | ISBN 9781774032435
   (softcover) | ISBN 9781774032442 (Kindle)
Classification: LCC PS8569.A429 B44 2022 | DDC C811/.54—dc23Email: info@silverbowpublishing.com
Website: www.silverbowpublishing.com

To all those
on their final journey
... heading home.

A Silence of Echoes

Sadness:

A scream
held in a silence of echoes.

The colour of a tear
held in a snowflake.

No artist could paint
what flows through my fingers
like ice.

Contents

Those Gone Before / 15

Aging / 67

Transitioning /119

The End? / 189

Those Gone Before

Behind The One Way Mirror

They Live.
They do live on,
in that other hazy dimension,
just beyond our reach.

They walk.
They still walk
the canyons of our minds,
turning memories on and off,
in cinematic film clips of days
past, present and future.

They dance
to their own rhythm,
feathers
brushing against our being,
echoing...

> *'Remember me.'*
> *'Remember me.'*

They breathe
their presence into our souls
to fill the empty space
they left in us ...
when they left us.

We live.
We do live on
behind this one-way mirror,
just beyond their reach,

> *Waiting ...*
> *Waiting ...*

for the mirror to shatter.

Dried Flowers of Youth
for Rex Howard, 1930-2012
BC Country Music Hall of Fame inductee 2004

Dried flowers of youth crushed between pages.
Forgotten utterings of ancient sages.
A whisper and scream and the drama between.
Life unravelling at the seam.
A young man running through early chapters
hobbling toward final ever afters.

You leave this world more every day.
Slowly you're slipping and sliding away
into the nether land of yesterday.
And oh, that I could follow you there:
To leave behind this worry and care.
To build with you castles on the beach
in that world you visit when you're out of reach.

Whispers and memories of your sweet song.
When you were young. When you were strong:
Before the years made your bones ache.
Before your hands started to shake.
Before you had to be wheeled in a chair.
Before time left you nothing to spare.

Dried flowers of youth are crumbling now
gracing the stage in their final bow.
Your frailty of heart will soon set you free
and far, far you'll fly away from me
to a place where roads are paved with gold.
Where dreams cannot be bought or sold.
Where music never ceases to play.
It will call softly and take you away.

And as you leave this world behind ...
the best part of me will become undefined.

Remains of the Day

Time and time again, I recall:
My mother's warm, yet vapid atmosphere
encircling me,
while somehow
still holding me at arms' length.
The uncertain smile
that tugged playfully at her lips
then disappeared
as quickly as it manifested.

So many years have passed
since I've heard her voice,
but sometimes, I swear
I hear her calling my name ...
in soft velvet whispers.

      In dreams,
   her voice calls
in louder tones.

There are times,
when out of the blue,
the pungent scent of her perfume
wafts into the room,
lingers for a few moments.
then disappears, but not totally.
A fine, filmy residue
of that moment
remains and gives way
to the fine, filmy residue
of her ghost.

Time and time again,
I linger in the past
holding onto her memory
and... the remains of the day

And I Knew

I saw my mother sitting in my living room,
and where she sat the living room was aglow,
becoming a sparkling light,
emanating all colours of the rainbow.

She did not see me watching from the staircase.
A mirror image tangled in the broken spokes of time.
Slowly she moved from shadow to starlight.
As I stirred to move toward her,
dew's cathedral opened to the yawning rose
she held in her fragile hand, glistening,
within the ancient reflections of my soul.
Her shadow, stretched out before me,
began to diminish and fade,
My own, in established disobedience,
dissolved into a river she could not swim.
She turned in slight confusion.
I heard the uneven beat of her heart.
The atmosphere thickened.
Strange mahogany doors,
bolted closed with platinum locks,
rose up and flew open as I knelt in awe.

Under a glittering crystal chandelier,
I saw my mother haloed in an amber aura.
I stepped into the golden embrace of her flame,
and my mother wept for me.
Stripped to the bone, standing immortal
in her shroud of tears,
sunlight and ice bound her eyes
into frozen cameras and sliced her tongue,
so, she could not speak of the sins
she had witnessed laying at my feet.

A tear fell.
Her ghost dissolved
into the thick of the atmosphere.

The exhaled breath of the night
composed her simple eulogy without words.

I saw my mother sitting in my living room
        and I knew ...
                she wasn't dead.

Mother

After I kissed your cheek
I turned my cheek
as the tears shivered
rivers of aching pain
into my wrist and fingers.

I was crying for you
and I was crying for me.
So many years together
and yet, so much time apart.
And now you were flying away forever,
a beautiful bird
leaving me behind.

I saw the glint of silver,
shining on old memories,
sparkling, for a moment in time,
as did we before our time was over.

Now, a new kind of lonely,
     Emptier.

Not a day or night will pass by
when I don't think of you.
Not a smile or a tear will appear
without some image of you in it.
You'll always reflect in me
like a deeply rooted diamond
dusted and powdered
with the sweet, salty, sugar
of yesterday's dreams.

And now,
I am orphaned;
but the mother and child reunion
is only a motion away ...
     Only a motion away.

22

Spirit Mood and Tone

There is a spirit mood and tone
in the smooth of this grooved evening.
A remembering of things
hazy and forgotten
lost in a veiled past
that invades this heart
with a palpable knowledge
of lives past, loves lost
and those missing.

On the road to tomorrow
the journey is more lonely
at the depth of a star,
shining on two people long ago,
melting their spirits together,
tethering their essence
with a fine silver thread.

      Unbreakable!
      Suddenly remembered
      like coveted raindrops on the tongue
      after a long, long drought.

There is a spirit mood and tone tonight
invading my being on every level.

I see us,
so near, yet so far apart,
and I shed a tear:

      Remembering things forgotten.
      Remembering you.
          remembering me.

The Dream

You walk in dark shadows
at the edge of night
and softly climb into my dream.
And then the music plays.

We slow dance
through the notes,
writing love letters on suspended chords
as we tap our way into each other.

There is a silence of voices throughout
as we search to find the lyrics that define us,

> side-stepping searching for
> the keys we lost.

As I grasp for them
they dissolve at my touch.

You fade into the dark shadows
at the edge of night,
climb out of my dream
and the music stops.

I cling to the silence
seeking solace,
trying desperately to re-enter the dream,
knowing full well I can't.

You Take Me by Surprise

Walking,
breaking into a run,
chasing my ghost
down the corridor of crimes
I committed against myself
in the name of something
I thought was love.
Trying to find it again,
yet praying I won't.

Turning the handle of the road,
I step back into a rough rain
scratching down my cheeks,
a hard ache squeezing my heart.

You always take me by surprise.
Your ghost creeps into my mind
on sleek nimble feet:
Walking past locked doors with no keys.
Gliding through thick concrete walls.
Entering the womb of my want.
Nuzzling the seed of my need.

When I least expect you,
your spirit wraps itself around me,
a pure wool blanket,
scratchy and abrasive,
yet somehow wet and warm
on the skin of a cold memory.

An unexpected guest,
you take me by surprise ...
always.

Between the Thin Pines

I see you walking toward me,
between the thin pines,
dimensionalizing into my realm.

You are frail and old.
Dressed in a blue plaid,
worn and faded, cotton robe.
You are smiling a questioning smile
right into the core of my existence.
You seem so small between the thin pines
dotting this enormous emotional landscape
we stand on in this dream ...

If I turn my head your image fades.

I close my eyes for a minute; then open them
and see you growing taller between the thin pines.
Looming larger and reaching out to my spirit
with your desire to be with me again ...

If I turn my head your image fades.

I close my eyes for an hour; then open them
and see you standing beside me.
Close enough to touch, but still, just out of reach.

And I don't know what to do.
You've been gone so long, so permanently,
with no possibility of coming back.

But you have come back.

And I don't know what to do
because i did carry on without you
into a new life and now, here you are
wanting everything to be just like it was.
But that was then ... and this is now.

And I don't know what to do ...

> *So, I turn my head,*
> *the dream dissolves,*
> *and you fade from view ...*

into the impermanence
between the thin pines.

Grass Quilt, Stone Pillow

Under his grass quilt
and stone pillow
he sleeps wrapped in his own silence
in dunes of weightless snow,
on starry nights filled with light.
His eyelids are closed
but still, dreams of his lover
invade the shade of his lost yesterday.

A capsule of love's living blood
dropped from her hand
not long after his last breath dissipated
in her mouth, her heart; but not her soul.

Lying on his stone pillow
he rustles beneath his grass quilt
opens his eyelids and whets his lips.
He will wrestle any devils
that may stand in his way,
that may come to give him grief.
He wears his invincible heart on his sleeve
and climbs out of his death into breath.

In the still of the night an escort of angels arrives,
in a flurry of wings, transporting him to her side.

His head sinks into her eider-down pillow.
His heart sinks into her sleeping spirit.
He kisses her gently; holds her forever
then vanishes into the last vestiges of night,
back to his bed in the dark wet soil
　　　　... where he waits.

Under his damp grass quilt and ice-cold pillow of stone
he casts a kiss to the wind and prays she'll feel it,
damp on her cheek, when she awakes.

The Ring of Death's Sting

I've lost my edge
in synch with the fading essence of my perfume.

    I am half-sleeping beside the television,
one eye peeled open,
    watching all the stations at once.

        In the corner of my mind
            a jukebox starts to play.

       In the ring of death's sting,
       there is a hollowed-out static
       in a rolling ocean of subtle sound.

    I wait for the gap between beats,
    which I know must inevitably come.

              I wait and wait.
         I am half-asleep
       wrapped in this limitless silence.

    Then the telephone rings.
I answer it
        grasping at straw dogs
    on broken leashes
        hoping to hear your voice once again,
      hoping to hear you say,
            "It's all just a bad dream".

But it's not you,
        and I'm caught
       in the ring of death's sting,
       and I've lost my edge
       in synch with the fading essence
            of your after shave,
      and ...
    you're never coming back.

Angular Circles

The days pass by in angles and circles,
jagged edges and smooth trails
as I travel to somewhere,
losing this,
misplacing that,
on the way to tomorrow.

Highways, roads, pathways
leading toward,
leading away,
travelling blind
through back alleys of disguises
in a shape shifting landscape
of microcosmic errors.

I journey on
through diminishing years:
recalling smiles and tears,
days of roller skates, wagons and bicycles,
riding full circle back to myself
on the broken wheels of yesterday.

In this moment of grooved silence,
my indulgences and iniquities rise up
in shredded flags of unconditional surrender:

Mistakes,
roads not taken,
memories I never made
still haunt me.

I wander the angular circles of my mind
in a never-ending maze.

Sometimes I see you there,
and I smile through a tear.

Before Your Eyes Closed

You were
my world.

My sun rose and set on only you.

You were
my moonlight.

My dreams turned to gold inside your embrace.

You were
the brightest star in my sky,

spilling dust on my heart to warm it.

The last time I saw you
I held your hand
and looked at you hard with love

I saw the story of my life
written in your eyes
before they closed.

Every Day

Every day
I visit that little corner of my heart
I keep you in.

Every day
I shed a new tear
for an old memory, embossed in gold,
that bears your name.

Every day
through life and death
I'll visit that little corner of my heart
I keep for only you.

A part of you
        will always live in me ...

                        always.

Fifty Years Later

She walks into the sky.
He finds her with a knowing eye.
He's been waiting so long.
They approach each other
fifty years later.
Time ceases to exist.

Her hands, gentle and loving.
The horse's breath, warm on her cheek,
tendrils of life,
slicing the early morning crisp.

He balks slightly at the bridle.
It's been so long,
but he remembers
its cold steel weight.
Its pinch.

She whispers to the steed,
calms him, tosses the bridal aside,
grabs a handful of mane,
swings onto his powerful back
and feels his haunches
quiver, tense and respond
in excited recognition.

Knees anchored softly
against his sleek muscular shoulders,
she feels their bodies become one,
the way it used to be
fifty years ago.

No longer horse and rider,
now a gliding machine
slicing through timeless time
and the brush of wind.

She sees the familiar ditch approaching.
Did he still have it in him to jump it?

Her belief in him flows through her loins
into his loins.

His gallop quickens.
His power shifts into high gear.

They glide over the ditch effortlessly,
rider and mount
fused together forever
in that beautiful moment,
the same moment they jumped through
fifty years ago.

Now,
never again to be parted,
they'll race with the wind forever
and the wind will always let them win.

Fluid Silence

There is a fluidity to this silence,
a timeless tango,
dancing to the whisper of a familiar song:
The strong, silent type.
Tall, dark and handsome.

There is a flexibility to this fluidity:
Slow to rapid.
Vapid to deafening.
Spinning,
within its own harness.
     Dangling
          on a string.
Thinning to a thread.
Quickening to rope.
     Encircling my thoughts
          in its net.

The same familiar song.
The same timeless face.

I always waltz with you
     through those lost hours
          in the warm hold
             of my fluid silence.

Dream

All my days have been a dream
unravelling at its tattered seam,
spilling inglorious indecisions
onto vague nights and indistinct visions,
chasing the moon past the edge of the sun,
watching the spectre of stars come undone,
reshaping a whisper into a scream.
All my days have been a dream.

I'm but a shadow in a dream.
Professing that which least I seem
I stand amid the fog and gloom
beneath a raging sky of doom.
I hold within my aching palm
the residue of sorrow's calm
where doubt and hope criss-cross and creep
in seas of heartache hot and deep.
My eyes are burnt I cannot weep.
I'm half awake but still asleep.

The echo of a midnight gasp
fades in words I cannot grasp.
I watch the light of day elapse.
I see the dream I am collapse.

I stand unravelling at the seam
inside this dream within a dream.

All my days have been a dream ...
                just a dream.

Hollow Gasp

We are:
> droplets of water,
>> the dust of stars,
>>> the breath of angels.

We walk
> through this pretense of reality,
>> this fabrication of truth,

> trapped
>> inside the dictum of our youth,
> flying
>> through fantastic space
>> as the world spins and spins.

We are:
> flakes of snow,
> shards of ice.

>> locked inside
>> the hollow gasp
>> of death's death,

>>> pirouetting,
>>> dancing
>>>> in and out of time
>>>> with timeless time

>> in a never-ending pool of
> timelessness.

We drift and dream,
> again and again,
>> inside the dreams we create,
>> inside the dream we are.

Knowing

The inky sky spreads,
    stains the windows of the train,
        obliterates the tear-stained face
            peering through the misty window.

    Time passes.

The horizon swallows the train.
    The sky engulfs the horizon.
        The night slowly drowns
            in the dissolving moments
                Of endless time.

    I melt into myself,
        one last time,
            this side of heaven's clock.

    Beneath her broken hands
        and bruised faced,
    I stand in the clutch
        of a relentless rain.

        Knowing,
        deep in my heart,
        you're leaving ...
        and
        I'll never see you again.

Obituary

And soon my heart will beat no more.
And long I'll be gone from this world.
Unseen in a realm of seen things.
Unreal in the realm of reality.

Long ago and far away
in the young days of my naive youth
I thought I wanted you.
Thought I loved you.
Puppy love.
Unrequited.

Slowly in those young days
I came to terms with the fact
you'd never be mine.

Years passed.
Our paths crossed slightly
only three of four times.

Quick, stilted conversations.

Somehow, we always were uncomfortable
around each other
and still, I don't know why.

Maybe it was because
I was uncomfortable with myself.

I read your obituary the other day
and wondered
about the life we never lived.

Beyond the Shadow of The Veil

Beyond the shadow of the veil
of themes and dreams and schemes,
we walked our roads with grace and ease,
and sailed on stardust seas,
then it was done, and we were one
and we will always be,
hand in hand beneath the sun
together flowing free.

Present, future falling fast,
into living moments past,
we'll live inside each other's breath
where there's no never-ending death
Where all roads lead to love,
by grace of God above.
Where mountains beckon us to climb
to the pristine edge of time
safe within each other's hold
where dreams cannot be bought or sold.

And we will love each other more.
'Twill be again as 'twas before.
My heart handcuffed by your kiss.
Your heart shackled to my wrist.
No separation will exist.
Love so strong it cannot twist
but strong enough to bend.

My lover and my friend
from time's inception to the end
beyond the shadow of the veil

A Hint of Perfume

After your death
there was nothing left of you
for the longest while.

I imagined
        the sound
of your voice speaking to me;
        you calling out my name
                from somewhere far, far away.

Years later,
        alone in an empty room,
                I would sometimes smell
                        a hint of your perfume:
                                Immediate.
                                        Pungent.

                I would turn and scan the room
                        for a hint of you
                        but I was still alone.

As years pass by,
        alone in an empty room,
                many times I suddenly smell
                        the scent of your perfume.

                I still turn and scan the room
                        for some trace of you
                        but I am alone.

I know you're not there,
                but ...
                        I've come to realize you are.

The Veil

There was an ambiance to the evening;
an atmosphere,
    a thinly veiled succor,
        a sugared honey
             from the Garden of Eden,
     glazed over the sweetness of the moment
that passed s l o w l y
        over the lips of the night.

    A summer rain
        fell from a pale blue sky
           as the wind grooved
               to the surreal
                       u
                  b   m
                           p

          and grind
      of the raindrops.

There was an ambiance to the evening
    thick with your imagined whispers
      and misty touch.

        ... I almost felt the veil.

This Slight Rapture

There always remains
at least one left over spark
        or ember
to light the darkest night

  and there's always
  one left over memory
to soothe a broken heart,

I stand,
romancing the hands of time,
to fly the painted kites of yesterday
high in a summer sky again.

Wrapped in my solitude,
swaying with the rhythm of the fire
and dancing in the rapture of a tear,
I feel your breath on my cheek
momentarily.

Always there remains
a hint of your after shave,
and an image of you in my mind,
permeating this slight rapture.

A Wisp of Haze

I heard a weary voice inside my head.
A wisp of haze and then your body rose.
Magnificence shone on the ghostly dead.
You stood oblivious in silver clothes.

You did not notice me as I stood there.
I tried to grasp your hand but it dissolved.
You sat down in your favourite easy chair.
A wisp of haze and then the room revolved.

Old memories flew round like mockingbirds
that brought with them a few unwelcome strays.
I saw you move your lips in silent words
before you disappeared into the haze.

Tonight, I'll wait for you to reappear
inside the hardened edges of a tear.

The Blue of a Fading Song

Trapped in the Blue of a fading song
another long night lingers on,
the music and the dancers gone.

I'm lost on a street of shattered dreams
unravelling night at its tattered seams,
searching for an ember or spark
to light my way out of this dark.

Then a sudden moon rises above.
Little stars sparkle like bright eyes in love.
Twilight flexes its fingers and reach
enshrouding an empty, desolate beach.
A seagull's cry slices the sky.
An empty teardrop falls from my eye.

Trapped in the blue of a fading song,
with notes and chords that don't belong,
I stand at the edge of a broken seaside
bathed in mystery and moonlight,
searching for you and yesterday
and distant dreams so far away.

Another long night lingers on.
The music and the dancers gone.
They've disappeared into the dawn
        but I remain,
trapped in the blue of a fading song.

Ship Of Dreams

My ship of dreams has tattered seams
    and rigging torn and frail.
A broken mast of memory's past
    shoring up its sail.

    And all the live long while
        no measure of a smile.
No consolation gleaned from happenstance.
        A brief romance, a passing dance,
    in cold fell clutch of circumstance.

    All the days, a drifting haze.
    The dimming of lights. Nondescript nights.
    Years pass like fog, wet, waterlogged.

And later, on some golden pond
    your pale ghost may arise
        to shine your smile into my eyes
            and take my heart beyond
        the earthly confines of this life
    away from heartache's pain and strife
where we can drift on ship of dreams
    seaworthy with tight seams.
        A mast of sturdy elm
            with two hearts at the helm
        and love that cannot fail,
    shoring up its everlasting sail.

        I wait here in my ship of dreams
        tattered at the seams
    wishing on a distant star
        and wondering where you are ...
            wondering where you are.

The Strand

Yesterday
     a wet sun spilled diamonds and pearls
          onto the sparkling strand.
             The wind caught our hair
        and took our breath away
    as we walked the beaches
of another place for the last time.

Today,
     there is no sun.
       I am a statue
          turned to stone,
       standing alone on the strand,
    far from the beaches we walked.

On days like this,
     I try to envision your face,
         but you've been gone so long
    your image is hazy.
I try to tap the days of old
     and dance within their crease and fold,
         but they escape me like a lost breath.

And now,
     the windblown day is swept away.
        A brittle silver moon rises
     spilling zircons and rhinestones
onto the shadows on the shore
     and the statue on the strand.

        The day
       and the strand
        dissolve ...

    as if they never were.

Beautiful Butterfly

The butterfly followed me along the shoreline.
A beautiful butterfly of colorful design.
How odd, I thought, on a day so hot,
that a butterfly would follow the blue water line.

It started to flutter to and fro,
with every step, each stop and go.
Mostly drifting on my right-hand side
as I walked the shallows of the incoming tide.

As the day grew weary and I traveled on
I thought that butterfly would be long gone.
But, alas, it steadfastly stayed at my side
as I walked the shallows of the incoming tide.

I walked and I whispered to that butterfly
of memories and dreams and days gone by.
I was certain it was more than a mere insect
as it seemed to command my deepest respect.

And then it hit me out of the blue.
Perhaps it was Karma and someone I knew.
I began humming a familiar song,
a hint of your essence sidled along.

A beautiful butterfly followed me home.
I knew you were here. I wasn't alone.
Now each day I walk along the shoreline,
my beautiful butterfly soft on my mind.

Empty ... Full

My heart is empty
     behind its blood smeared walls.

A pale ghost
     walks the canyons of my mind
whispers through my veins
tries to reach my heart.

I can almost smell his after shave
and feel his breath on my cheek.

The sound of his song
echoes faintly in the caverns of my care
and I weep inside its haunting rhythm

     His voice whispers
          in the falling tears
     softer than the tears
yet louder than any other voice that invades.

Today
     my heart is empty,
        yet still full ...
           full of yesterday.

Fistfuls of Moonglow

Carrying fistfuls of moonglow,
      I walk through the star dusted streets
            with the dead that come to my door.

They swim effortlessly
      through the dark waters of time
            seeking the cool of my winter blue eyes
      as they cast off the heat
            of summer's stale embrace.

They are the masters of black fire
      and indelible indigo flame.
            They shine in shards of mirror
      reflecting kaleidoscope years
            pouring memories and dark water
      into the heel of my heart.

Carrying fistfuls of moonglow
      I lay at the altar of the lost
            near the crossroads of death.

I leave the star dusted streets,
with only the imprint of my footsteps
      in the fading drops of moonglow
            as the dead dissolve in the mist
               whispering,
         almost inaudibly,
               auf wiedersehen.

Gathering of the Trees

In the gathering of the trees,
I romance the tears of an old June moon
  to coax dead memories to come alive.

Just beyond the Poplars,
  underneath the Elms,
    a ring of bright water and sparkling stars
  are creating a beautiful melody
that rises in torrid notes
  to dry the tears of the old June moon.

There is a clearing in a channel of the sky
  and a nearing in the stardust on high
    as I rest in the gathering of the trees
  in the midst of old June moon memories.

The ring of bright water and sparkling stars
  pull me into their magic
    and the whisper of your voice
  tugs at my heart
    and sings me back home again.

This Quiet November Evening

A white dove nested in a net of stars,
     a dark raven caught in a sea of tears,
       and all the while
the rain ripples and runs
     beneath the veil of night,
creating a brand-new pool
     to reflect the age-old stories
that lay resting
     in the lines on my face.

     This quiet September evening
wears a jagged teardrop pinned to its breast
     as it turns the blurred pages of my life
     and weeps for me again and again
     at the end of every chapter.

There's an ache in my chest,
     a tear in my eye
     and a hazy familiar memory
        riding tall
     through the dimly lit canyons
of my mind.

     Always...
       always it's you.

Familiar Star

In a tangle of barbed wire and frozen flame
I heard you calling out my name.
I saw you standing across the bar
in the glow of a distant familiar star.

I heard a faint whisper echoing afar
from the glow of that familiar star.
So, I deftly began to cross the bar
to yesterday's kiss ... to where you are.

And then a loud noise broke my dream.
Your ghost faded into a misty moonbeam.
It all seemed so real and you seemed so alive.
I looked at my clock. It was 3:45

In a tangle of barbed wire and frozen flame
I swear I heard you calling my name
in a faint hazy whisper echoing afar
from the glow of that fading familiar star.

Heaven's Arms

Dancing to a memory long since gone,
like a haunting song you linger on.
but somehow I've forgotten all the words.
They've flown away like lost hummingbirds.

But still, I hear that distant birdsong.
It whispers to me as I walk along
old trails and old familiar places
where love gently put us through her paces.

Although you're gone, sometimes you seem near.
I feel your touch, turn, but you're not here.
Each day I leave this world a bit more
As I inch ever closer to death's door.

And if I chance to stand inside God's grace
I fancy when I pass I'll see your face
And each lonely year and tear will fade
As I lay down to rest in your warm shade.

Dancing to a memory long gone
I still hear that distant sweet birdsong
Then suddenly I'm standing in God's grace
I hear your voice and I see your face.

You are the music and I am the score.
We'll sway in heaven's arms forevermore.

One Heartbeat Away

I'm dry inside this falling rain.
Time and 15 streets away,
these age-old streets connect again
in shimmering long ago display.

I spy a lovely butterfly
with glistening wings, passing by,
and oh, that I could fly to you
and turn our yesterdays anew.

I close my eyes and move through time,
through music, rhyme and pantomime.
I see you standing in the light
glowing in the dark of night.

You're only one heartbeat away.
I want to come, but I must stay.
I hear the sound of Earthly things:
Children's laughter, playground swings.

And so, reality steps in,
I'm back inside time's Siamese twin.
You're only one heartbeat away.
I long to come, but I must stay.

One kiss and one embrace away.
I long to come ... but I must stay.

Stallions of Time and Tide

You are always with me
      riding high behind my eyes
          speaking in gentle whispers
            only I can hear.

The sacred butterflies of heaven
      fly seamlessly
          through the gaze of my eyes
     and gather in the shade of my heart.

I don't have to close my eyes
              to see you.
     You're indelibly imprinted
            onto my being.

You're always with me
      riding high behind my eyes
          on the stallions of time and tide.

Laying Soft Upon My Heart

A glimpse of steel, a flash of train
silent on an endless track,
and oh, that I could ride again
the rails and not look back.

You still waltz across my mind,
a tender wistful melody,
and in those moments lost I find
the music brings you back to me.

We travelled light with heavy hearts
and rusty throats that could not sing:
Victims of our own false starts,
Dragging winter into spring.

And now the years have come and gone
since those days spent on the road
We've travelled light years from our song.
Days grow old and nights are cold.

But still, you waltz across my mind,
a mellow Monet work of art;
and in those moments lost I find
you laying soft upon my heart.

A mellow Monet work of art ...
laying soft upon my heart.

The Days of Old Gold

I carry old, tattered photos with me
from yesterdays etched in my memory.
There's a picture of us in a blue cabaret
and instruments on stage we used to play.

I carry lost days in the back of my mind
and I never know when they'll start to unwind.
The old days are with me wherever I go.
You're still in my soul ... I want you to know.

The days of old gold have come and gone.
They've faded away like yesterday's song.
Winter's arrived with gray clouds and rain
and the days of old gold won't come again...

No, the days of old gold won't come again.

Slice Of Rain

I stand in a slice of rain,
damp with yesterday's tears.
Your face hazes in and out.
Eyes that never dry,
follow me everywhere,
burning me to the core.

Blood and ink stains
wash over my spirit
in this storm that never subsides.

Standing in this slice of rain,
I am never alone ...

Your image is everywhere.

The Funeral

I stand silently,
outside the reception hall.
Ashes to ashes.
Dust to dust.

Death is all around.
Cold in the earth.
Warm, walking on the concrete.

You're gone never,
yet forever.

We, the remaining, exchange:
Tears.
Faces.
Smiles.
Embraces.
Compassionate words.

You, the departed, remain:
A footprint on life's water.
A ripple on the earth.
A whisper on the wind.
A tearstain on the ocean.

Indestructible!

You're gone never,
Yet forever.

Rest in peace
little one...

The struggle is over.

Solace

So many autumns
come and gone,
shuffled into a fading sunset,
caught in the chill of winter's breath
and the eternal sorrow of my mind.

So many faces and voices
dimmed with the passage of time.
Acquaintances forgotten.
Lovers only slightly remembered.
        Save one.

I find solace
in the whisper of your name.
In the imagined touch of your fingertips.
In the seasons of yesterday
overlapping all my barren todays,
all my tomorrows,
all my sorrows.

Some Days

Some days
　　　　　I am afraid to die.
On these days
　　　　　I am more careful,
　　　　　　　more alive,
　　　　　　　more extravagant.

Some days
　　　　　I am not afraid to die.
On these days
　　　　　　　I am world weary,
　　　　　　　　　brow beaten,
　　　　　　　　　anxiety riddled,
　　　　　　　and contemplating
　　　　the luxury of a quicker entrance
　　　　　　　　into the endless sleep.

Some days
　　　　　are jeweled beaches.
Some days

　　　　　are damp gray sandbars.

The days pass by in a daze.
　　　　　The nights dissolve in a haze
and I find comfort in my maze...
　　　　　　　some days.

Down to the Sea

I go down to the sea
to the lonely sea
where I know I'll find you.

I walk as fresh paint
brushing against breeze and tide
onto the canvas of time.

I listen to the spill of the ocean
as it tries to get into my eyes,
my heart and my soul.

I always start
from the lifeguard tower
at the west end of the beach
and end up somewhere
that seems like a pre-destined
destination I should be at;
where I'm sure you're close by.

You're gone but you're here.
I'm here but I'm there.
The real is surreal
and the surreal is real.

I go down to the sea
to balance my heart and soul;
to balance the here and hereafter.

I go down to the sea,
to the lonely sea ...
where I always find you.

You Are Here

The gentle toss of the breeze
through my hair,
whispering kisses onto my cheek,
dries the tears in my eyes
as I picture you still here beside me.

Sweet Prince of time and tides,
you roll in gently
onto the shorelines of my mind.

I hold hands with your ghost most days.
Today is no different.
I feel your gentle caress in the wind,
your warmth in the sun's embrace.

I see you so clearly
sitting on my right.
It's unimaginable to think
you are not here,
so, it must be true.
Somehow,
you really are here.

Background voices filter in
beneath the whisper of your breath.
You are here.

You are here
with me always.

There is no death.

The Still

After the rending apart,
the cracking of the rose,
the wilting of the stone,
a bony finger
scratching at the soul
claws and clings.

Tears, still damp,
on glazed blue eyes,
shine and roll
on iridescent waves
of remembrance.

An immense stillness
creeps in, pervades
where your silhouette's fingerprint
still emanates a cloyed essence
of bittersweet root and stale mint.

              In the echoed atmosphere
              of the still,
              a branch breaks.

        De Profundis!

      A raindrop falls.
    A melody whispers...
          and I wait
    for the music to start.

      I wait for you.

Aging

The Aging Process

One day you'll understand
why my mind is somewhere else
when I seem to be looking through you,
or into the edges of the mirror or the walls.

Every day I walk a little slower,
laugh a little softer, ache a little more
and carry yesterday's kisses and wishes with me
in the fragile cradle of my heart.

You may notice me searching
for words or something I lost
long, long ago in the keep of my youth.
My mind wanders deep inside old memories
and tears brim in my eyes much easier
than they did yesterday when I was young.
Even now as I write these simple lines
tears are sliding down my cheeks
and I know not why...
I know not why.

I find I'm thinking of old days,
old friends, and old loves
that disappeared so quietly
but are not forgotten.

Sometimes I can't recall their names
and their faces seem hazy and blurred,
but their words still echo in my heart.

Sometimes I close my eyes.
Dreaming awake, I see their faces, hear their voices
amidst a glow of music playing softly;
and I imagine I'm dancing again.

I've come to realize this is the aging process...
One day you'll understand.

Waiting Room "A"

The scribble on the whiteboard stated:

Welcome to waiting room A.
Black writing glared from the oval mirror,
stark but welcoming in its own way.
It put me at ease and quelled my fear.

Five others sat in the cold waiting room
lost in their thoughts inside the gloom,
anticipating what their next test would show
inside their private riptides to and fro.

One thinking on better days gone before
she ended up here by this waiting room door.
The woman with the long brunette hair
was coming undone and just sitting there.

A little blonde girl by her mother's side
shared a look of love that could not be denied
as the man in the hat, at the end of the hall,
stood up to answer the technician's call.

Staring at the mirror in waiting A
I thought of results that would soon come my way.
It's all in the cards and the luck of the draw
dictated and subjected to karma's law.

In the Akashic records it's written in stone.
We enter and depart this world alone.
None of us know how long we will stay;
or when we'll be summoned to ...
                              waiting room A.

Before the Stars Can Shine

I watch the evening sunset expire
in the chokehold of another dying day.

Dark honey drips
from the flayed fingers of night
blotting out the last remnants of light.

There is an inferred whimper,
a muted whisper
and a moment of total despair.

But always ...
always there must be darkness
before the stars can shine.

Early Morning Haunting

Through the foggy lens
of an early morning haunting
the ghosts of summer,
windblown voices
and hazy dreams
still linger
in the blue shadows
of a dying star.

A pearl scarf of frost glistens
under a red rising Sun.
A lone gull cries to the wind
leaving its imprint
in the thick atmosphere
of a muted October sky.

My footsteps crunch and crackle
on a scatter of pebbles and leaves
that whisper secrets
into the outstretched palms
of this early morning haunting.

I watch the sun rise.
Ash to ember to flame.
I listen to the wind.
Silence to whispers to voices.

I'm alone, but not alone.
I walk with ghosts
in the blue shadows
of this early morning haunting ...
                                    haunted.

Hollowed-Out-Crack

Is this stranger in my mind a hologram?
Is this real or just a dream?

I am viewing myself inside out
through the hollowed-out crack
of a one-way mirror.

Locked inside a fractured mind
and screaming soul,
I wonder ...
where is the spirit hiding?
Why did it loosen the ties that bind?
And what will become of the pieces of me
so carelessly scattered to the winds of change?

On the cutting room floor
of my backstage film production,
none of the pieces fit the puzzle.

I am viewing myself from outside in
through the hollowed-out crack
of a broken smile.

Passing Things

Sometimes I hear voices and noises
                that nobody else hears
        and I wonder
                if it's the other side
        reaching out to gather me into their fold.

Sometimes I smell a waft of perfume
                and I swear
                        my mother is nearby.

Sometimes. I swear I glimpse a ghost,
                a fading grey shadow
                        nudged into the corner of my eye.

And there are times
I recall a jig-saw puzzle memory
                with a few missing pieces ...
                        or pieces that don't quite fit.

These are passing things,
                passing fast,
                        then slowly fading away ...

                                as am I.

The Stardust of Bygone Days

Plastered against a pulsating horizon,
    the ageless faces of friends and lovers
        dance and romance
           the fading stardust
              of bygone days.

    A pale silver sky
        turns to gun-metal gray,
           burns to charcoal,
        then to dark bituminous night.

        And still the faces
           parade through the shade
        of my star dusted aging spirit.

Drunk on the taste of yesterday's wine
    I toast the flavor of today
        and the faces fading away
           into the ghosts of the past.

    I relish the last few sips
        of life's bittersweet wine:

        One last look at the empty glass
           and I fade into the stardust
        of all the days gone by ...

           and I become
           endless night.

Unbound

I try to recapture
        the lost, almost forgotten joys
                of childhood days and ways.

      I try to marry them
           to an aging heart
              and failing mind;

The pictures in the photo album
                have yellowed.
        The glue has lost its stickiness.
        The book of life
              has lost its bind:
        The pages kidnapped,
            are imprisoned
        in the inner sanctum of my soul.

      And I am becoming ...
                unbound;

        fading, fading ...

                fading away.

Turned Inside Out

Wandering into Alzheimer's night
I'm fading away from reality's light.

I've forgotten the words to your favourite song
and the lyrics to mine don't seem to belong.
I can't differentiate between right and wrong
and the memories I cherished are now lost and gone.

I reach for my cane as my hands start to shake.
I can't recall when my bones didn't ache.
I look in the mirror and see a white streak
has replaced the black strands of my widow's peak.
Then my mind starts to wander. My eyes glaze over.
I'm a child again running through fields of clover.

But still there are things I barely remember
and January's now just a prolonged December.

These things I've learned from my sojourn on earth:
There are two sides to everything: each of great worth.
A whisper's the other side of a shout.
And today is just yesterday turned inside out.

My Name

Slipping in and out of consciousness
        and this recurring dream,
I search for the missing objects I've lost
        along with the letters of my name.

I travel the shadow of my soul
        trying to unravel the pages
            that used to be me.

I'm standing amidst my baggage,
        without a destination
            begging a passerby
                to take my hand
        and take me to the land of lost alphabets,
            that I may find my missing letters
                and know my name again.

Burnt Embers of Death

These words are aglow with an inner fire
    spilling from the depths of my soul.

The roses of hope
    I tended so tenderly
        have died once again on the vine
    with no chance of a resurrection.

The burnt embers of death
    have turned to ashes
        and crumbled to dust
    in the dead of the killing night.

I remain with the remains:
    a bittersweet painting
        of burnt embers ...
    burning out
        lost without a compass
    on a stone-cold ocean of ice.

        I'm slowly drift, drifting away
    on the bittersweet winds of change
        and the surreal burnt embers
          of death.

The Forgetting

I forget things now with a bit more frequency
        followed by a hollow feeling of alarm,
                but there is a comfort
                        in the forgetting.

                It wraps itself around me
      a warm blanket, a lullaby,
                    and for a moment I'm a baby again
        in a flash of dream and sleep.
              then back to reality
        which seems a more unfamiliar fit
              with each passing day.

        The aging process
                needs the forgetting
      to prepare us
             to leave the familiar.

I forget things more and more,
      with each passing day,
            as I cling more to my warm blanket
                in the unfamiliar lullaby
                    of my last chapter.

A Frozen Tear

In the solicitous hold of a crescent moon
I sigh on a beach of star kissed waves.
I am the nadir of midheaven's peak
etched onto the passage of nondescript years.

And I long to talk to the trees again,
To walk barefoot and free on the beach
back to the roots of the me I lost
so many distant moons ago:
when everything old was new again,
when every dream lost was found,
and every wish I tossed to the wind
had a chance of coming true.

But alas we can't go back ...
time is shivering, standing still
and I am a frozen tear.

Water and Rain

I long to go down to the shore again:
to hear the water speak to the rain,
to see the seagulls fly on high,
to hear the sadness in their cry.

The tender years when I was young,
when rainbows 'round my shoulders hung.
Those sky-blue days of golden tears.
These sky-blue eyes long for those years.

The long and winding path grows pale.
The mast now hung with ragged sail
sits all alone on a desolate shore
and I'll hear the seagulls nevermore.

The fleeting magic of youth is gone.
Life's music now a fading song.
The sky-blue skies have turned to gray
and soon my soul will fly away.

The days of life are beginning to fade,
an age-old stain on invisible suede.
And I long to go down to the shore again
to hear the water speak to the rain ...

to hear the water speak to the rain.

Page of Life

Moving across the face of the sky,
a paint brush
and fingerprint
began to write my epitaph.

It was later than I thought.
I had been sleeping
at peace in the bed of life
unaware of the rapid passing of time.

Drifting and dreaming
to the beat of my heart,
wasting time
on a glittering neon street
where words came aplenty
and life flew by
like a flightless bird.

As I looked up from my papers,
the ink was fading fast from the page.
The finger writing my epitaph
had disappeared
and the ink was almost dried
on the last line.

I saw myself slipping and sliding
on the tears of regret,
stumbling
and fading, fading
from the page of life.

Sky Pastels

I gaze through the windows of my soul
at the sky pastels unfolding ink blots,
periwinkle and blurs of turquoise
smeared against the afternoon sky.

Unframed paintings of moving still life.
Monet dreams dreaming,
setting the scene.
for what dreams may come

I sit,
somewhere between my signature
and the half-written page,
watching the ebbing dusk
flow into the hard-edged corner
of a crystal twilight star.

I see the world dim
in slow motion fade out
as I sign my name
to another day...
passed away.

Watershed Moment

In the sparkle and shine
   of the china cabinet walls
     the porcelain and crystal
       glisten and glow.

There's a feeling of yesteryear
   spinning around and around
     flooding the crisp atmosphere's
      moody overtures.

Images stumble
    through the mirrors of my mind
  and wind
     through the backroads
     of old memories.

    I see a horse standing alone
    at an empty water trough.

I see a wingless eagle worn to the ground
beneath a crumbling ledge of tears.

I slide off the sparkle and shine
   in my eyes.
  into the watershed moment
    of the here and hereafter
  and the dull-edged glint
    of reality's blurred sword ...
  and the drowning begins once again.

Overhead

Dull, wet, clouds sleep overhead.
A droning ebbing and flowing
permeates the neap tide of passing traffic.

I see pedestrians and vehicles
zigzag between the raindrops
    and each other
in a quest to get somewhere
    that really is
        nowhere special,
    and yet they rush
in the crush
    of car and human,
        tides of flesh and metal.

I continue to peer,
    through the mire of skin and tire
        trapped in the wire
        of life's ring of fire.

    Half alive and dreaming
        half asleep and dead,
    I am a ghostly puppet
        hanging by a thread.

Dancing with dead stars
in the shadow of the sun
    and the whisper of a hush,
    I slowly come undone
        below the sleeping clouds
      sighing
      overhead.

Inside the Thinning

Between the thinned firs,
a small pale-yellow house
sits encased and slightly visible,
between the faded brown trim
of the surrounding trees,
lodged inside the sparse of winter.

There seems, still, a hint of sparkle
beckoning to a long-ago sun
hiding in a crease of cloud
in a forgetful sky above.

Inside a thinned crowd of people,
I am an insignificant figure,
hazing in and out,
encased in the capsule of life,
a captive of my flesh and breath.

There seems, still, a flicker of light
beckoning me back to my past
to tap the crease and fold
of the long-lost days old.

In between life and death,
        I remain,
    aging, lessening,
        trapped ...
    inside the thinning.

On the Horizon

A distant haze crowds in on the horizon
and some clouds look like they have suits and ties on.
It's a whimsical, imaginative world today.
The kind that makes your heart want to play.

So, I'll pick up my cane and put on my shoes.
I've got nothin' to lose but these little town blues.
So, out the front door then at a snail's pace
I pass a guy on a scooter in my own senior's race.

I wait patiently for the light to turn green
Then check for right-turners if you know what I mean.
The old guy beside me says in a drawl,
"Driver's today! I don't trust 'em at all."

I watch where I'm stepping so I don't trip and fall
on this crumbling sidewalk that leads to the mall.
I do my shopping as quick as I can
then get in the line-up to pay the sandman.

That's what I call him 'cause he's slow as molasses
as he squints an peers through his pop-bottle glasses.
Always making mistakes and wasting my time,
I curse to myself in resigned pantomime.

With my bag in my left hand, I head to the street,
cane in my right hand and shuffling my feet.
I see some clouds still have suits and ties on
as I head toward the haze ... on the horizon.

Lilac Butterflies

Long, long ago,
      beneath a muted twilight firmament,
I once sat with the lilac butterflies.

      Their fluted wings, bolts of shot silk,
          glistened in the satin glow
              of a silver neon moon.

      A cool rain fell in vanilla dreams
cascading softly onto summer's poetry.
      I laid nestled inside its pages,
          turning the seasons inside out,
      while the lilac butterflies twitched and trembled
          inside their dark purple dreams.

Then one ice-chilled day ...
      a raw, renegade wind
          scraped at the silver neon moon
      slicing at its face, cutting it to the quick
until its luminous cheeks turned crimson
          then purple,
      and the lilac butterflies scattered.

Tonight, caught in the cloyed crease
      between yesterday and today,
          and hungry for days gone by,
      I will walk the desert sands of my heart
          beneath an aging twilight sky
              trying to recapture
          the lost lilac butterflies of my youth
      with my tarnished magic wand
and my tattered net of poetry.

A Cold Flame

A cold flame runs through my dreams
      burning a tribute to the ashes
         that hold the history
            of all my lost yesterdays.

      They blow through the canyons of my heart
         echoing the music and the name
of someone I can't remember.

I bump into non-descript shadows
      trying to find that heat I recognize
         that fire I once was.

I shuffle through the images in my mind
      trying to find that crease of time
         I became lost in.

A cold flame runs through my dreams
      burning a never-ending tribute
         to the music
and the name
         of someone I can't remember
someone who died ...
            but is not dead.

A Spring Too Far

Wandering through this place I should know,
the once familiar signposts
      dotting the now treacherous landscape
            have become blurred
      and unreadable
            in the fogged climate
      that continuously invades
            my days and nights.

The summer winds have faded.
      The autumn leaves have fallen.
        The chill of winter
            is too cold this year
               to hold any promise
                  of spring.

      Wandering around,
        lost in this place I should know
            but don't recognize,
        I stand in silent hope
            wishing for
          and dreaming of
        a spring too far.

A Thousand Voices

The question has a raw, red edge
and the answer has a thousand voices
            that ping and ring
            through the land I am.

I try to construct a sentence
            of music, song and angels' breath
            but the consonants
            asleep in the vowels
                    are losing coherence
            in the saw-edged corners
                    of my disappearing syllables.

            and though I know
        a thousand voices ring and ping,
            the only voice I hear is mine.

Alone and Anonymous

I sit quietly disoriented, beside you,
    alone and anonymous.

    Drifting into a new dawn
        the fog of forgetting
           has invaded.

        I look at you now
     through a distorted tear
  and see only
another stranger.

    Alone and anonymous,
      I close my eyes
        and quietly re-enter
        my own lonely space.

Faces, People and Places

So many faces,
        people and places.

        the familiar faces
    are becoming unrecognizable
    and the unknown faces
    seem strangely familiar.

Flowing forward and backward
    on waves of transitional time,
        I swim in a sea of confusion and sorrow
    and slide down the tears of the years.

Then suddenly,
    someone steps out
        from the wheel of transitional time
        and burns the blur off my haze.

So many faces,
    people and places,
        all familiar strangers
    sharing one thing in common with me:

        none of us know who I am.

A Solace of Sorts

The skin of my soul
is cracked and dulled,
hanging loosely
on an ancient amber shield
that's war weary
and seen better days.

Emotions flash and bend
like elastic starlight
stretched past the point of return.

Mirrored smoke in my mind
rises, forms hazy images
that look like someone
but resemble nobody I know.

Weakened by the frayed threads of time,
        I sit silently
within the faint thrum of my heartbeat.

I stretch my skin taut
over its tarnished amber shield,
      seeking not redemption
          but a solace of sorts.

A Time

This is a time of ebony moonlight;
A season of ice-cold sunshine.

I walk
on blood white trails
in a burned-out ancient forest.
Ashes stir and swirl
in a torrent of mixed emotions.
Branches flail at my heart,
cindering my soul,
blurring my vision
to the colour of truth.

       Shadows and rocks
       melt together
       on this precipice
       distorting my view of yesterday.

In the grand expanse
of the eternal now,
this is a time
of unmitigated consequence,

       A time ...
I wish I didn't have to acknowledge.

Lost Water

Alone and afraid,
I cross each smile
with a tear.

Depression
is miles above me now.

I am the lost water
of a desert dream ...
   dying of thirst.

Phantom Dance

The sky is a dazzle of starlight.

A hard rain spills,
in punches and jabs,
onto hollowed out deerskin and bones
that decorate my barren house of stones.

The wind whirls and swirls,
hums and drums.

I am aware of many phantom voices
inside the citadel of my nights
where I dance with ghosts
inside a forgotten song.

Just a Daydream

In a hospital room on the 2nd floor
I thought I heard a creaking door.
Strange rooms and beds make for strange noises.
I'm imagining whispers from strange voices.

A burgeoning fear manifests as sweat.
A foreboding feeling of impending death.

I'm stuck in room 210 on the 2nd floor,
But it's just a daydream and nothing more.
And I am a daydream and nothing more
dreamed by the dreamer minding the store ...
A daydream ... and ... nothing more.

Sometimes I Dance

In the barren courtyard of my mind,
    sometimes
        I dance
           to remember.
              Sometimes,
            I dance
            to forget.

      I dance alone
but always I dance with you

There is a bittersweet haze
    wrapping its arms around me
      whispering
    in a seductive, raspy voice
            You can stop dancing
             anytime you want
            but you can never leave
Day by day
    and night after night
             the dance lasts
          longer and longer
      Day turns into night
    Night turns into day

Through the haze,
    I hear my phone ringing.
        It just keeps on ringing
          and ringing
      but I can't answer it.
      I'm lost in the dance.

Sometimes,
    I dance
   to remember.
        Sometimes I dance ...
           to forget.

The Rhythm of the Universe Within

A hard rain claws at her eyes
and tears at her ears with harsh words.
Electric metal robots
and wristwatches that don't work
are her only companions in this den,
this invisible forest she's dancing through.
The melodies are timeless and torn.
The rhythm of the universe within ...
> *sighs.*

This den should be crowded,
but it echoes with her breath only.
The rhythm of the universe within ...
> *cries.*

The melodies have lost their soft edges.
They're dissolving into
stumbling notes and broken chords,
unaware of the key they were written in.
Timeless and torn. Old and worn.
The hard rain continues,
but now in whispers she can no longer decipher.
The rhythm of the universe within ...
> *dies.*

She can't dance anymore
inside this crumbling steeple.

> She's lost herself
> and she's lost
the rhythm of the universe within.

> *She cries.*

This Ever-Prevalent Fog

It's been a hard day's life today
and an even darker night.

The stars don't shine anymore
Inside this ever-prevalent fog
I find myself permanently wrapped in.

I can't seem to unzip this night, and ...
the north star has gone into hiding.
My compass is broken and ...
direction has become impossible.

There's an anguished scream
lost somewhere inside me,
clawing to get out,
searching for a vacuum to explode in.

This fog crept over me
while I was sleeping inside a dream.
I'm awake now
but I'm still lost in this ever-prevalent fog.

    Directionless.
     AND –
I've lost the dream too.

A Deadly Splash of Green

There is dust on the sidewalk,
rust on the leaves
and a forest alive with a deadly splash of green.

I sit in a separate space,
beneath a dappled blue sky,
content in my makeshift tent.

I am a wayward poplar
surrounded by evergreens;
a cedar growing roses
on a desert dune of melting snow.

In the corner of my eye, I see a random tear
dropping from a weeping willow's aching heart.
In the edge of my ear, I hear a whisper
beckoning me deeper into the forest.

I start to crumble, like the ancient relic I am,
into the dust on the sidewalk,
the rust on the leaves,
exhaling my final breath
in a deadly splash of green.

A Pale Yellow Sky

A wayward star glistens
on the whetted lips of the breeze.

Across a pale yellow sky
a rising moon sits astride
the wind's coat tails,
riding slices of shadow
and shimmer,
spinning haphazardly.

I, too, spin haphazardly
on a torn and tossed renegade wind,
dissolving in the misty tears
of a dying sun
under the half-mast eyelids
of a pale-yellow sky.

    The sky and I ...
       both of us,
old beyond our years.

December Heart

Through a crack in December's air
a winter song claws its way into my heart
and my night coils cold again.
An ice-clad moon sinks
behind the clouds in my eyes
in the dust-riddled gloom of the room.

My weary eyes peer
through their scarred lids
at a parade of unknown faced
        dissolving inside
the wounded atmosphere
        I reside in.

Through a crack in December's air,
        night coils colder
  around my December heart
inside this winter I can't escape.

Sides

Outside

        the sky bends down
        to kiss the ocean.

Inside

        my shadow flees from the light
        into the land of endless night.

I stand

          beside the empty chairs
          inside the lonely room
            waiting
        inside a dim forgetful silence.

Outside

      a waxing moon
      shines the ocean's face.

Inside

        the room and I shiver
        inside the crushing loneliness.

The Gap Between Pulse Beats

I understand the gap
between pulse beats.

This is the playground of ghosts
acting out dreams
in a one-dimensional landscape
beneath a quivering ocean of sky
that threatens to rain
in a blue stain of tears.

There is a depth and pressure
to the rough stubble fabric
of tonight's thick atmosphere,
and a razor's edge to twilight's glow.
There's a curl to the wind
and a twist to the barb-wire clouds
slicing through the heat of the night
scattering embers onto the moon
searing the cross of a star too far.

I understand the gap
between pulse beats

This semi-death that has not yet been stretched.
This space in between feels no different
than the echo of the pulse.

When it stretches to infinity
we will know the full embrace of death
and we will see there is no difference
between life and death
but simply a long-exhaled breath
and a gap in pulse beats than never ends.

This is the place where death dies

I understand the gap
between pulse beats.

In Broken Pieces

On wet gray days
clouds blanket a slow-moving sky.
Rain murmurs in small tones
like damp petal flutes and muted violins.

On nondescript days
mist clings to the trees.
Its ghostly fingers flexing,
caressing the creeping twilight.

On dim charcoal nights
fog clings to the broken edge
of a buried sun
reflecting a shattered sky.

On nondescript nights
the moon hides behind damp clouds.
Stars shimmer then disappear
into the panther's paw.

Minutes and hours
parade by in broken pieces
like unsolved jigsaw puzzles
the texture of exhaled breath,
the colour of an unnoticed death.

On wet gray days
alone feels lonelier.

She Waits

Perched by the window,
she sits waiting,
watching,
listening
for that which may never come.

She searches spring rainbows,
hot sultry beaches,
glistening ski slopes
and listens to autumn leaves rustling,
whispering secrets she can't quite hear.

Suns swing high and low.
Moons masquerade by.
Days dissolve.

Perched on the edge of her bed
she is sleepy,
ready to dream
of that which may never come.

She grows old
in the cold hard breath of loneliness,
but still...
she waits, ever vigilant,
watching and listening
for that which will not come.

Blazing January Snows

I lay,
on the black nights
of an unwanted summer,
alone, keeping vigil
over a creeping damp.

I feed,
on second hand dreams,
smoky fireplace feelings,
wasted ashes,
and silent smoldering suns.

I am searching
for ice cubes
in the middle of July.

When the season has passed,
I will seek out flames
in the blazing January snows.

Discontent

A white lovebird,
flying in the sky,
delves farther into the purple haze
becoming invisible.

White clouds are in evidence
eating up purple patches of air,
chasing the sun
into a distant corner of the universe.

The mountains,
are vague blotches
on the fog-riddled horizon:
Not silver.
Not blue.
Not white-capped.

They loom in the distance
like disappearing islands.

It's less relaxed now.
Nothing seems to be at peace
Inside this looming discontent.

     Somehow ...
it makes me feel more comfortable.

Almost

All the houses I've called home
have crumbled to dust.

The sidewalks I once walked
are cracked and buckled now,
and somewhere behind that dead hedge,
beneath the bare branches
of the age-old broom tree
I played in and on as a child,
is the still beating heart
of a dream I could never lay to rest.

I can still glimpse little chunks of it
            glistening and gleaming
in tiny shards of stained-glass mirrors,
        hazing in and out at the core
of a rainbow city I never visited
                or lived in.
                Or did I?

I am
Almost
two people
becoming four, six, eight, ten, eleven,
but really only one ...
becoming none.

All the house's I've ever called home
have crumbled to dust
            almost
        like they never were.

                Almost...
            like I never was.

Wallpaper Fog

The afternoon
sprawls over dusty streets and sidewalks.
Dusk falls in pale gray tendrils,
ink spilling off papyrus,
shawling the shoulders of night
atop the weary day.

A wallpaper fog creeps in.
It inhales the voices of the night
        digesting them
into suffocated whispers upon whispers,
layering them into prayers
that have no meaning,
in this dense void of shallows
and undefined shadows.

        The wallpaper fog
      hangs damp and dingy,
        a bruised plum
      draping the edge of night,
        shrouding my world
        in razor sharp whispers
      of dreams that will not come.

Secret Shade

I'm fighting sunlight
and burning
in the freeze
of my thawing torment;

and so, death evolves,
a luminous fear
in the dark cavern
of its most secret shade.

Absence

In the absence of all,
beneath the big blue tent,
clouds drift and scramble impatiently
fleeing across a vast expanse of sky.
Night claws its way over the edge
    spilling ebony ink;
staining and fading the blue.

      Alone on the path
    I search for another set of eyes
      in this semi-glow of dusk.

Somewhere,
there is water
scrubbing the back of a warm beach.
Somewhere,
there are sheep
wending their way home
under the weary gaze of a good shepherd.

Here ...
there is only bruised sky,
blue turning purple, turning black
in silent right of succession.

By the time it reaches me
another set of eyes
will be impossible to find.

      I clasp my hands together
        In the absence
        Of one to hold.

Statue

An old guitar
        with broken strings;

   Music
        with no score.

    I stand
    inside my loneliness,

       a statue,
       nothing more,

The Step

In this painting
dawn spills from the rising sun.
The stars run away with the moon.

A white dove circles
above a black satin, slow moving swan
with far away eyes.

Black ebony swan
on turquoise glass lake.
White ivory dove
in azure silk sky.
The stark contrast
too beautiful to be a lie.

I step into this painting
and become real
in the tunnel of another time,
the echo of another universe.

I spill down
onto the stars and moon
and chase the sun away.

One step beyond ...
          become the dark.

Transitioning

Water Colour Sky

Falling, falling:
     Faraway tears from a distant dream.
Held in the saw-edged palm of a scream.
     Splashing onto a water colour sky.

      And somewhere
   at the edge of this world,
I know a new day is waiting.

A waterfall roars
    into the misty atmosphere
of a fading song I can barely hear
   or recognize.

    Slowly I reach for my guitar:
     Strumming
          the strings,
          the air
     and the moment
            onto the fingers of time.

    Whetting
          the dried, chapped lips
          of a memory
    to sing the faraway tears
           into a brand-new melody
    and sew the soul electric
           to the water colour sky
    and onto the fabric of now
where I stand patiently waiting ...
    somewhere
in between the seconds and minutes
     of then.

22nd Street Again

It's twilight time in the rain
at 22nd street again.

Somewhere there are golden sands
waiting on my lost footfalls.
Somewhere there are summer winds
beckoning me with soft calls.

And all the while I see your face
drifting through a sweet daydream.
And somewhere in the moving haze
the past unzips at the seam.

At a lonely bus stop in the rain
I wait to hold you once again.
I bide my time with bated breath
on the other side of death.

I'm pulled toward a soothing noise
drifting through the ether tide,
then I hear your velvet voice
and suddenly you're at my side.

It's 22nd street again.
The dark, you and me and rain.
Love still hums its sweet refrain
inside yesterday's ink stain.

We stand on sparkling golden sands.
The time apart now in the past.
I kiss your face and hold your hands.
The world dissolves; I'm home at last.

The Winds of Perpetual Winter

When the dark sky curls its cold arms
around my stiff glass body
and tightens its embrace,
there is a shattering of unseen emotions
that speak in hieroglyphs and tongues.

I can no longer safely guide myself
down this uneven, chiseled-out road ahead.
Too many twists and hidden turns above ground
and too many shifting sandbars and cities
submerged in the tangled kelp beds of life
It is no longer possible
to anticipate washed-out bridges
that lead to nowhere.

My heart sighs and wrinkles inside this glass body,
this glass turning fast to crumbling shards.

Behind the drawn curtains of night,
I sit in empty silence
beneath a blue, eclipsing moon

I think about the earth spinning slower every day
as the chains of death draw tighter and tighter.

the transience of life never so evident
as when the winds of perpetual winter
                    slide in
on the tracks of yesterday's tears.

The Final Collapse

I am a house of cards,
                words, music and dreams
       collapsing and resurrecting
             in new colour schemes.

       I'm balancing on the edge of a plate
       dining with destiny, supping with fate

I'm an aging house of well-used cards
         grasping for lost words, music and dreams,
         moving into the final collapse,
             coming apart at my ragged seams.

Death's bony finger is wagging and beckoning
       calling me to my final reckoning.

My house of cards is worn and drawn.
       I may not see another dawn.
The days grow short, so does my breath
       in the cloyed clutch of impending death.

Coming Undone

Dark sky shadows
on the mountain,
in the forest,
on the water.
A feeling of emptiness flows,
splashes and crashes
against the slick black day.

Inside this cold, I hunker down.
Knowing the frost and ice will come.
Knowing I am out of season,
past my *"best before date"*.

Dark age shadows
on my face,
on my body,
in my soul.

A reticent tear emerges,
flows, streaks and runs
into a wrinkled corner of my mouth.

Dark sky.
Dark age.

I've grown old
inside this cold.

I turn to frost,
then ice,
and finally ...

I come undone.

Dust on the Doorstep

Memories ...
dust on the doorstep,
sundrops on surreal patio lakes,
wind slicing through blades of grass.

Fading perfumed days,
long gone from the atmosphere,
yet, still here,
still clinging
to the hush of the wind.

Memories ...
hazy images,
stories swirling in the dust.

Stories I thought I might become,
burning brightly for a moment
then floating away
on a weather-beaten birch bark canoe.

Drifting
at the edge of my mind.

Fading
into the horizon.

The wind picks up speed
as the memories,
and my footprints
disappear ...

like dust on the doorstep.

The Book Re-opens

Tides, coming full
      yet waning and ebbing
            on fading shorelines,
      footsteps treading softly
      leaving their imprint
            on the pale blue iridescent dust
      of ancient skylines
as the waters of life embrace us.

      Wandering through cloud drifts
      and mother of pearl pyramids,
      the days shine amber
      against opalescent nights.

      Years, ages, faces,
            tears trading spaces
                reverse through each other
            spiralling the seasons,
      riding the rivers of life and death.

Windblown pages always moving,
                        forward,
            backward,
    opening,
            closing,
                going past the end,
back to the beginning.

Through the pale iridescent dust of infinity.
Through the sparkling waters of eternity.
Onto the wheel of karma and rebirth:

      A wink, a sanctified blink
      and the book re-opens.

Frost on the Grass

Quiet mornings pad in on tiny mouse paws.
Stillness pervades the silence
as dawn trips over the darkness,
chants adieu to the fading moon.
It's winter, cold and lonely,
wrapped in a blanket of mist.

Afternoon atmospheres hang heavy.
The windows are painted with frosty figurines
dropped from nature's icy fingertip.
             Some seem familiar.
A few melt into orphaned teardrops,
fleeing, in search of a warmer tomorrow.

Nondescript evenings loom large
on the stage of ebbing light.
A hazy dark clings to the edge day,
swallows the dissolving twilight.

             Now, in this late season of my life,
             I look at everything differently.

Yesterday dialogues whisper,
echoing in the silence,
ebbing and flowing softly
through disappearing star dusted nights
and cool crisp mornings fading,

             The season and I
               disappearing ...
             like frost on the grass.

Crumbled to Dust

Hands, now icy cold, crumbled to dust,
once coursing with blood, warmth
and the fire of creativity,
deftly crafted this fine piece of Coal Port China.

Did this gifted artisan laugh too loudly?
Love too deeply?
Did he don masks to hide his tears
and wear paper smiles in public?
Or did he weep openly,
parade his scars for all to see
on a stage of his own making?
And was the stage solid
or did he build it on weak and shifting sand?
Did he give one too many performances?
Or did he leave them aching for an encore?

As he gasped his final breath
did his hands feign applause
as they lay limply on his chest?
Or did he feebly try to wring them in angst?

Registration number 91750,
this piece of fine coal port china
remains locked in life's prison.
The hands that crafted it have escaped
on the wings of the angel of death.

I remain incarcerated in life,
eyes fixed on this ornament,
very much aware of my hands
soon to be icy cold ...
crumbled to dust.

Dead Stories

Dead stories:
chained to necklaces of grief,
emerging from the dark abyss,
wash onto shores of the living.
They whisper to me
of monoliths and pharaohs,
minstrels and poets,
lovers and losers.

Once alive and vibrant,
now awakening from the endless sleep,
silently cradled in a cosmic sea of dreams,
they wait to be born again
into fresh new chapters,
grasping for that first breath
of crusty satin air,
changing into the tight flannel
and cotton clothes of life,
becoming living stories
filled with familiar secrets,
writing new beginnings and endings
day after month after year
sigh after smile after tear
imprinting the atmosphere
with inspiration, passing away,
becoming dead stories once again.

They wait patiently in the womb of creation
for the still small length of a shortened day
in this universe of ever revolving dead stories
waiting to be born ... over and over again,

Dead stories
lying in wait to greedily grasp
that coveted crusty satin breath of air
                                    once again.

A Dream in a Dream

I have laughed like water
    and cried like dust.
        I am least what I seem
        in this dying dream:
    an iron maiden turning to rust.

There are songs I will never play
    and words I will never write;
        music I will never hear
        until my angels reappear
    and slay this cold hard night.

Life's just a dream, in a dream,
    softly sighing and crying.
        An altar for smiles and tears.
        A platform for joys and fears.
    Just a dream in a dream that's dying.

    Just a dream
        in a dream ...
            dying.

A Distant Moaning

A distant moaning:
a silent song, a wordless rhyme,
drums whispering a broken lullaby beat.
The dead dance to their own music.
They dance to the songs only they can hear.

A string of pearls.
A chain of golden silver.
A pendant of burnt amber.
A candle of sage and sienna.

These are the things
that remind me of the dead.

These are the things I will take to the dance
when I hear the distant moaning
and move slowly across
Time's river of tears
toward the dance of the dead.

A Matter of Punctuation

It comes down to a single moment
cloned from a bit of history,
from a box inside a box, inside a box,
where my poems are layers of skin
hidden inside my bones.

The birds of silence have landed
with broken wings
and taken up residence inside
the ever-changing hours and minutes of my mind,
where the seconds keep winding down
past the limits of the faulty metronome
that has become my life.

I still have my words
and a vague memory of a haunting song
that plays like a rain dance
stolen from an indigenous dream.

I imagine the movements,
supple and static,
as I mime the names of the dead
for no reason at all except
to pay tribute and respect.

Tears punctuate my sentences
and form rivers in my story
as it heads toward the silence of the lake
I know awaits just around the bend;
and suddenly there it is.
The flowing story of my life
and the lake that holds
all my punctuated sentences.

And there it is ...
The end. Period.

The Understanding

We are knee-deep
in our own patterns of eternity
weaving the destiny we wear,
mapping the world we create,
stumbling through dreams,
tripping on nightmares,
cutting our teeth on the knife of life.

Visible and invisible,
peeling hours like oranges,
sharing slices of time,
we are ghosts
filtering in and out of sky and soil.

Dreaming ... we're lying awake.
Awake ... we're inside the dream.

We are the vapid expectations
of our own personal poetry
filling page upon page
with fog and sunlight,
moonglow and stardust.

      Waist deep ...
we begin the understanding.

Dimensionalization *(a sonnet)*

Could I be but a structured form of paste?
A hologram believing I exist?
A spirit in a hybrid state of grace?
In actuality just moving mist?
Am I a portal to the other side?
Or mortal merely biding, chiding time?
My spirit's breath can never be denied.
Its perfect rhythm interlaced with rhyme.
My structured form continues changing face.
This body's shed upon its final breath
as time and fate recycle inner space
revolving through the doors of life and death.

Dimensionalization blurs my eyes
as soul moves from disguise to new disguise.

Alone

I

Alone In the bourgeoning hush of night
there's a clatter and rustle of leaves
in the autumn equinox of my mind.

I am the aging mirror of my childhood,
a glint in the crease of elusive dreams
where every street is an avenue
and the avenues are forever.

II

Evenings alone,
in the dark of my own making,
semi asleep, hazing, dimensionalizing.

Days alone,
in the heart of my privacy
skipping stones and gathering shells,
remembering the sound of waves.

The edge of dreams an illusion.

III

Never far from those days
I walk down yesterday's lane,
alive with shadows and light,
which I'd hoped would follow me home
and warm the lonely evening chill ...
        so lonely ...
                so full of loss...

            ALONE.

Blue Mirror

There is an essence to the blue mirror
      that haunts the quiet of my soul
where hazy dreams become much clearer
      and sparkling diamonds are hewn from coal.

It's like stepping into another dimension
      and swimming in a cosmic pool
where there's no ebbing or ascension
      inside a warm and vibrant cool.

Inside the essence of the haze
      everything is crystal clear.
We spend our hours in life's maze
      on this side of the vast blue mirror.

With angels moving to my side,
      the blue mirror is beckoning me
to step onto its static tide
      and sail the waters of God's Sea.

As I move in and through the blue
      the mirror warms me to the bone.
I shed my flesh to walk with God.
      Nevermore to be alone.

Deep Inside the Dream

Cradled in the womb of time
I'm swaying on a quarter line.
I walk this dream with hobbled feet
down a dark and dusty street.

Beneath a brackish crescent moon
I watch twilight crash into noon.
I see the ornate cable cars
climbing to embrace the stars.

> *And all the while a silent song*
> *whispers as I travel on.*

It seems a quite familiar tune,
reminds me of a night in June
when I was summer in the fall
so far removed from winter's call.

> *And now the days are losing light*
> *as I hold hands with pending night.*

Cradled in the womb of time
soliloquizing pantomime,
soul unraveling at the seam,
I am the dream ...
        deep inside the dream.

Heaven's Sea

A distant water beckons me.
Close but still too far away.
I lie beneath a tall oak tree
and listen as her branches sway.

I visualize your tears and smiles
hazing through the fog and rain;
and I would walk a hundred miles
if I could hold you once again.

Inside the harkening twilight
a lonely whisper beckons me:
To walk into the waiting light.
To sail with you on heaven's sea.

Amongst the lilacs where I lie
I offer them my wettest tears;
and all the while the fading sky
above me slowly disappears.

No need to walk a hundred miles
to hold you once again.
I taste your tears and feel your smiles
Beckoning me into the rain.

I leave behind my written words,
my paintings and a melody.
I shed my flesh to fly with birds
and sail with you on heaven's sea
       for all eternity.

The Soft Strum

A silver guitar gleams in the moonlight
pressed to the lips of a star shining bright.
There's a mystic shroud draped over the night
and a song being born just out of sight.

The clock is ticking. It's half-past eleven
and I'm dreaming of you this side of heaven.
I patiently wait for the door to swing wide.
Two steps forward, one back, then inside.

The silver guitar has beckoned me here
from behind the veiled drape opaque and sheer.
The band is playing a sweet melody,
our favourite song for just you and me.

So, I side-step the storm and walk into the light
and the glow of angels just out of sight.
The music always brings me to you
on the soft underbelly of roses and dew.

Then every gray sky turns to baby blue
as I lie in the soft strum of me and you.

Songs of the Past

The sweetest songs of the past
            have long since been digested
                        in the echoes of lost time
      and I am sequestered in the moments of life
            counting the seconds and minutes
                        at the expense of the hours.

      Whispers and sounds of the future
            try to weave their way
                        into my ice-riddled eyes
            that I may see the future,
      but I am oblivious to the incoming tide.
            Unaware of my impending demise.

                  Oh, for that last sweet draw of breath
      before I dance again with death
to those sweet, sweet songs of the past
      long since digested
            in the echoes of lost time
      where I come face to face with myself:
            The real me,
                        The spirit I am.

I turn my ear to the quickening sound
            of those sweet, sweet songs of the past
                        softly calling me home.

      I reach out to clasp
            the welcoming hand of death
      and softly whisper through glistening tears,
            take my breath away ...

                  take my breath away.

The Sparkle of a Distant Star

Under the sparkle of a distant star,
a piano solos in soft blue notes
writing scripture on the air.
I walk along a pier of dreams
above the waters of an ebb tide.
beneath the blur of a pale, bruised sky.

    Reflections,
    ebbing, flowing.
reverberating down a rabbit hole
    into the nothingness
    that leads to everything ...
where I am part of the drifting haze.

The silence in never-ending and thick
    yet, somehow, I still hear your voice,
vibrating on a violin string,
    slowly becoming a chord,
      a melody,
    a song in the emptiness
      leading to everything.

I will follow the sounds
of the violin and piano
to the sparkle of that distant star
    that leads to everything ...
    that leads to where you are.

When All My Stories Have Been Told

In the crystal mirror of my mind
I watch the dream I am unfold.
I see my breath upon the air
writing stories to be told.

A distant bell is ringing,
a flock of angels singing.
I'm inside a living poem.
At last, I'm finally coming home.

We all walk through this world alone
on streets of gold or tarnished stone;
and as we walk our hearts begin
to turn to silver or to tin.

We all walk in the noon day sun,
moving snapshots on the run.
A footprint in the sands of time.
An exercise in pantomime.

I'm sailing an outgoing tide
heading for the other side.
Again, I'll hold hands with my soul
when all my stories have been told.

The Cross Over

I'm at rest in a dream of lilac and purple
as yesterday's waves are coming full circle.
They shine and reflect in shimmering grace
as I gaze again on your beautiful face.

So many years spent outside in between.
So many tears swept away and unseen.
It's time to cross over yet I must abide.
There's too many crosswinds and a riptide.

There's an ache in my heart that won't seem to heal
and things that were hazy are now coming real.
There's a needle pulling a thread for the dead
and I'm sorry for all the words I left unsaid.

The sounds of the world are fading away.
I have to cross over I know I can't stay.
I hear your voice calling from the other side.
A door in the sky is opening wide.

Death stands at the altar, and I am the bride.

I am ... the bride.

The Dance

Shall we dance?
    I ask that of the shadows
        that haze through my hazy days
            and haunt my dreams at night.

    I whisper to the wind
        and speak to the stars
        and then ...
            the music starts.

I stand at the sidelines
    back to the wall
        waiting for a chance to dance...
  a lonely wallflower
      on time's timeless stage.

    I am a shadow,
        a fading ink stain
            on the dog-eared page of life.

        Losing my balance
      and losing my breath,
    I haze and blend into the shadows
      and become the dream
        I am dreaming.

I let go of the last thread of life
        as it breaks ...
    then the music stops
        and the dance begins.

Grains of Time

I stand at the edge of a blistered moon
    watching the sand in the hourglass
        romancing the grains of time.

    I swing and sway
        on a dance floor of dreams.
          slipping and sliding
      across a river of tears.

    The storms of life
        blow colder today.

I stand at the edge of a darkening sky
    watching and the days of my life
        tumble down,
    as the last grains of time
        slip through the hands of life
          into the arms of death.

Highway of Stars

I envision a million miles
of finely sculpted and pebbled road
leading onto a highway of stars
while I lay lost and forsaken
on a beach of scattered dreams
that can never reconnect.

It's always dawn or dusk
and I can never find
the dimly lit pebbled road
leading onto that highway of stars
pre-destined to take me home.

I am baking and freezing,
caught in the cringe and crease
of invisible light and dark,
haunted by the absence
of suns, moons and stars.

Malingering on this beach
of promises cast aside
and scattered broken dreams,
I'm alive and yet dead ...
trapped in the fading echo of life.

The Scratch and Scarce

Inside the narrow wood
of pine trees poplars and birch,
I weave my way through the scratch and scarce
of scattered branches and bark.
The smell of a winter storm gathering
at the edges of the forest chills me
and I think on days gone by.

A cavalcade of hazy images
warms the frost etched onto my soul:
     summer beaches and wave-carved sandbars,
midnight bonfires and yesterday lovers,
     the sun swinging low on the sky's wrist,
a shiny bangle dusting the horizon,
     a harvest moon skulking in the shadows
     waiting patiently for its day in the sun.

There are pale ghosts hazing in the narrow woods
slicing through my eyes, whispering in my ears,
and there are echoes from ages past
still living and breathing
in and above the scratch and scarce
where season after season has fallen.

Here I walk, one last time,
beneath the sun, moon, stars and sky,
as the tender arms of the final winter
gather me into the scratch and scarce
of their haunting magnetic embrace;
then lay me down to rest forever
in the warmth of all my days gone by ...
     all my days gone by.

A Season That Never Dies

The autumn leaves drift and float down
      whispering to the river
as they kiss the songs of the dying season
      onto the lips of her tear-stained face.

This is the pale blue mirror of sky
      and the glimmer and glimpse
          of the living paintings
             moving and swaying
      beyond the shadow of the veil.

Inside this dream I am
      there is an echo of beautiful music
calling me home and home again and again.

Just like the autumn leaves drifting down
      soon I'll drift onto the pale blue mirror
         to reside with the living paintings,
         moving and swaying
         beyond the shadow of the veil
    to the songs of a season
        that never dies.

Voices of Yesterday

Today,
>> pale music from the past
>>> fills every room in my mind.

>>> Voices from yesterday
>> approach from all directions.
>>> The fading blue from my eyes
>> runs like watercolor down my cheeks.

In the mirror, I'm fading to grey, to pale, to invisible.

>> The full moon has fallen to its knees
>> and broken the fragile string of life.

Today,
>> I am sinking into deep water
>>> the color of pastel music:
>>>> a sweet serenade
>> sung by the voices of yesterday ...
>>> the voices I know so well.

Set

Such beauty and such horror do I find
when I delve through the canyons of my mind.
Unwinding and rewinding all my days,
I see the glaring error of my ways.

Looking backward on my distant past
I never built my hopes or dreams to last.
And now I shed a tear and breathe a sigh;
and now I live and now I'm set to die.

I'll say goodbye to all that I hold dear
as death's cold touch is drawing ever near.
I've lived and laughed and cried a little while.
Now no way back I've crossed the broken stile.

And now it's time to say my last goodbye;
and now I live and now I'm set to die.

The Tangible Dream

I carry my bones and flesh
through the broken chains of my life
searching for solid water
or a tangible dream I can touch.

Bewitching butterflies dance at my side.
Graceful dragonflies ride my neap tide.

Enchanting songs are chasing me down
a highway of hazy forgotten dreams
and I wish and pray I could stay
but the dream is fading and frays at the seams.

There's a distant whisper drawing near
in the lilac and jasmine of my mind.
where everything stops and comes full circle
to square the music to the score.

The dragonflies read
from heaven's scrolls
as the butterflies
cleanse my soul.

I shed my bones and flesh,
breaking the chains of life,
as I walk upon solid water
and embrace the tangible dream I am.

The Winds of Tomorrow

The winds of tomorrow tap and knock at my door.
I keep them at bay and don't let them in.
I'm on the last steps of the stairs to four score
and the essence of life is shedding its skin.

Staring out through a rain-stained windshield,
cold and alone sitting in the car.
I close my eyes and I'm in a green field.
strumming the wind with memory's guitar.

There's a girl in a pink dress on a park bench
with a black spaniel puppy parked at her side
and behind both of them there's a white picket fence
enclosing the graveyard where all my love's died.

My eyes are wide open though they remain closed
as misty figures come alive in my head.
Then from out of nowhere I see your ghost.
In the heart of my soul, you'll never be dead.

It's a cold day in January split at the seams.
I'm putting asunder all my old dreams.
The world is gyrating in a slow-motion spin
and the winds of tomorrow are fast closing in;
                              fast closing in
as the essence of life sheds the last of its skin.

The Stuff of Drifting Dreams

At the purple hour when my eyes turn to dusk
I see twilight dreams spinning through stardust.
leaving a pale purple trail I can follow
out of this graphic world empty and hollow.

And that's the way it sits. I'm really here, but over there.
And on my father's grave so cold, I honestly can swear
we are just drifting stuff made up of space and air:
Atoms, molecules and quarks and muons everywhere.

There is a screen we see them on
but when we look away, they're gone.
As we turn our gaze, in reversible twist,
they disappear. They no more exist.

We are the purple twilight mist
crumpled into night's dark fist.
We are the stuff of drifting dreams
falling through life's tattered seams.

Here, there and everywhere.
Everywhere and nowhere.

Blown away in the twist of a wrist
in visible, invisible mist.

We are the haze
and the glaze in life's maze.

We are only ...
only the stuff of drifting dreams.

Just Beyond the Gray

In the drift and grift of a gray afternoon,
waiting in the car beneath fir and elm
in the Saturday city parking lot,
a rustle of ghosts draws my attention.
A murder of unseen crows noisily announces
the opening of gates from another dimension.

> *It's so calm and serene,*
> *yet, otherworldly and eerie.*

And then through the din,
the gentle chirp of a robin
who has defeated the army of militant crows
with his tender song of peace.

The trees have fallen silent.
The world is almost asleep
but the robin and I keep vigil,
scanning the visible
for the invisible.

In the drift and grift of this gray afternoon
I sit quietly, caged in my solitude.

The robin continues to chirp,
slightly louder,
waiting patiently for me to follow
into the rustle of ghost ...
just beyond the gray.

Blurs And Smears

I am dying

     I can no longer fly.
     My wings are broken.

       I am becoming
       a smudged obituary,
fragments and bits
of shrunken soul
       that no longer fit.

        I am dying
      in the wake of decayed stars;

drowning in blurs and smears;
     a fading ink stain,
      undecipherable.

        Lightening cracks
        every time I die.

Ghostly Carnival of the Undead

I am lost in a carnival of the undead,
unable to find solace
in my heart or my head.

I'm dazed and confused
           in this circle of squares.
                I'm lost in this maze
        of crumbling stairs.

      A white band of skin on my finger
            is evidence of a past love gone by
               and sometimes I cry
                    but I know not why.

Broken lyrics
      loom large in my head ...
           Are these my words
                or words left unsaid.

      Is it rain from the sky
or a tear in my eye
      or a total breakdown instead?

          Try as I may
        I cannot escape
this ghostly carnival of the undead.

Hazy Shadows of My Ghosts

I ride the rails of my mind
        tumbling with the curve of the track,
stumbling, scattering onto a random landscape
        as the train whistle cries to the wind.

        A bright sky of blue sorrows gathers
and sheds tears disguised as raindrops
        onto my broken compass.

        The distant echo
        of the train whistle haunts me
        down to the bones of my soul.

My thoughts scatter
            at the turn-style of serendipity
        as I gather with the hazy shadows
            of my ghosts
        to ride the rails of my mind
        down to the soul of my bones.

Where the gathering meets the deep
        and I can fill my basket of need
        with baubles, bangles and beads
            and all the things I'll never need.

I Am

I am the pale ghost of the night
flowing through cobblestone streets
unnoticed by the lovers
hiding in doorways
and under the bridges of time.

I pass by pastoral gardens
and vibrant, living canvases,
painted with faces of long-lost relatives,
drifting on sepia toned gondolas
down faraway sleepy canals
that whisper familiar lullabies.

I have become one
with a sky without borders
closing in on my fading shadow,
absorbing my ethereal essence.

The faraway echoes of a timeless universe
pull at my hazy figure
as I drift above the cobblestone streets
not certain if I am dead or alive,
but certain that
                    ... I am.

Monochrome

There's a monochromatic tinge to my days
    that crept in on little mouse feet:
        noiseless, innocuous,
          on the slick sweat of death's breath.

I've walked through my shadow
      long, long ago
and traded places with a lesser me
    that stole all my cherished songs
      and left me empty
in a house of mirrored silence.

    And now,

the last remnants of colour
    are fade,
      fade,
        fading away
    as the monochrome turns to gray
      then black
      then nothing.

    And the mice slide away
      noiseless and innocuous
      on the slick, cloyed sweat of death's breath.

Residence

In this place,
where dead is alive
and alive is dead

your eyes
are disembodied sparks
burning the chaff off the dark edge
of this endless night I am walking through.

I am tangled-up in a timeless tango
of motionless motion,
silent sound
and disembodied sparks
exposing the shadow of your ghost.

This is the place
where dead is alive
and alive is dead.

This is where I reside.

The Far Tree

I gaze out the window
to the far tree across the lane,
bending and swaying,
a pawn of the wind.

I am unaware the sun is setting
rolling toward the fading horizon,
twilight chasing the light of day
into the edge of night.

I watch the far tree
and the dulling lane
disappearing into
a fast-encroaching purple sky.

I watch darkness, my old friend, descend
and zip the last remnants of daylight
into the pocket of night.

Stars twinkle through its threadbare fabric
and dust the edge of the far tree
to make its presence still visible to me.

At this moment
the far tree and I
are the only actualizations
in the midst of my world
slowly disappearing
day by day by day.

The Mirror

Words pass between us
and as soon as they are spoken
they dissolve.

Laughter is left behind
in a place I may never find again.

      I move closer to the mirror.
      My face looks slightly familiar,
      like someone I used to know

          I try to go outside myself
          to feel where I've come from
          and where I'm travelling to.

I search the shifting patchwork sky
for a brighter shade of this blue
I'm walking through.

Fingers of uncertainty
are strangling the blue
blurring it to gray
brushed onto the back
of the mirror I'm looking into...
and now my face looks unfamiliar
and I can't find
the road I must travel
to come back into myself;
and all my bridges have washed away,
and the mirror is dissolving.

Dream Creation

Through a foggy rainbow lens of possibilities,
    I search each prism and colour
        for the dream I created so long ago
            in the ether of another time;
          another place.

Somewhere there are flowers, pools,
    birds and butterflies
        that know the pathway
    leading to this dream I created
        so long ago.

    The flowers won't talk.
      The pools remain silent.
    The birds speak an unknown language;
        but the butterflies ...
     the butterflies know my name.
They whisper the way
    and wipe the foggy lens
      with the flutter of their wings.

I dive into the lens,
    through the prisms,
        melt into the colours
and become the dream I created long ago
      the dream I have always been ...

      the dream I am.

Liquid Stone

Sleeping on liquid stone,
the pink of night approaches
emerging from the womb
of a broken stone-age dawn.

It throbs and pulsates,
with forgotten songs
and blurred melodies,
leaving footprints on the water.

On the river's pale pink sheen,
a long-lost dream skates by
losing an edge
on the wheel of time.

Awakening to a stir of echoes
this moment caves in on itself.

The liquidity of life disappears
into the set of stone
slowly ...
slowly ...
becoming spirit.

Lost Dimension

I'm all alone,
in this nourish nightmare,
with no one to slay my dragons.

I find myself
in the company of a suicidal sandman
who won't part with even one grain of sand.
>He just keeps tossing more tears
>into my broken eyes.

I'm trapped in this temple I've created,
replete with cracked paint and crumbling walls.
>The ceiling is sagging.
Surely it will cave in on me soon
>and then,
I'll never be able to find myself again
>inside this lost dimension.

Lost to the World Again

Night rubs its whiskers
against my heart
chafing the edge of emotions
still red and raw at the core,
dead on the surface.
The wind cracks her knuckles gently
against the streaked window-pane
and I am lost to the world again

In the still small silence
of hazy memories
a hollowed-out whisper remains.

      A snowflake in summer.
      Liquid lightening.
      There for a moment.
      Fading like quicksilver
      into a stir of echoes.
      Vibrating.
      Dimensionalizing.
And I am lost to the world again.

Painted rain fingerprint stains
across a dark sky
are random yet repetitive,
forgotten yet familiar.

      I search them frantically.
        for the key to me.
      The key to set me free
          to be
      more there than here.

I drift away
on the breath of the breeze
and I am lost to the world again ...

      ... lost to the world again.

Melting Surreal Train Tracks

A drooping pale-yellow horizon
    melts into the surreal train tracks.

A bright navy-blue ribbon of twilight
    falls lazily across a fading summer horizon.

    The gray butterfingers of dusk
        slowly spread dark honey
            onto the sky.

There is a face
        in the window of the train.
    A lonely face:
        stained with teardrops,
        etched with a deep sorrow,
            grooved into a memory
            the soul can't recall
            and the heart can't forget.

In the window of the train
        there is a face.
            A lonely face
      watching a million miles
    of melting surreal train tracks
        slowly disappear
      into a fading tear-stained horizon.

Merging Dimensions

In the flex and fluid flux
of inter-dimensional tectonic shifts
laid bare on opaque plates,
I glimpse a multiverse of realities
laying within the crease and fold
of the *"Eternal Now"*,
of the *"I Am"* and *"The All"*.

The bone shifters and spirit walkers
quantum leap and skydive through merging dimensions,
dissolving boundaries
on the diamond-studded rim of reality's wheel,
spoking through paths of possibilities,
dancing at the edge of dreams,
spinning them real
on the continuous weave of the loom
inside the *"Eternal Now"*.

Out-picturing myself from myself,
I rest in the curve of an angel's wing,
in tune with strange melodies ...
Melodies that soothe the savage heart
and excite the spirit electric.

I dimensionalize
in cryptic silence
and golden hieroglyphs
into the vibrant hum of the universe,
becoming the rhythm,
becoming the music.

Fully dimensionalizing
into the merging dimensions
of the *'I Am'*.

Blending in surreal magnificence
into the whole of *'The All'* ...
        I re-merge.

November Fog

Through the cool of night
the fog and damp creep,
clawing and stroking
the edge of my mind.

On the wave of a tear,
a tiny memory
is gradually drowning
inside a hazy sea.

Under a golden glittering mallet,
I break glass snowflakes
falling through my thoughts
like miniature earthquakes,
stumbling and tumbling
over second-hand icicles.

A burnt dawn invades
a broken sky.

Melting in a silver thaw
I drip through the damp
and sink into
the hard-edged embrace
of a cold November fog
that somehow gives me comfort
as I travel further from myself.

Points

All my locations
have become unknown to me.
I am lost in the electric air
slicing through light,
scattering in points of darkness.

I am scorched earth
begging for the caress of rain.
I am freeze-dried emotion
praying for a silver thaw.

In the static of hollowed out sound
I pillage the night's exhaled breath.

Filled with the secrets of time,
I become a monolith of uncertainty
shaking within my crumbling foundation.
I'm searching for the key to myself
that I may scatter
in points of light in all my locations
and slice through the darkness
to sing the spirit electric ...
past the point of return.

Slip-Sliding Away

A sliver of silver moonglow
slides through
the crimson crunch of darkness
sewing the night
into a necklace of icy sequins,
encircling a lonely heart
laid deep in a pool of tears.

Where is the love that used to warm?
Where are the arms that used to comfort?

> Slip-sliding away...
> slip-sliding away.

Creviced between midnight and dawn,
stars have trekked into hiding:
Darker than black.
Blacker than night.
Thicker than sound,
muting the beat of a lonely heart.

Trapped in the clutch of a burnt-out star,
laid deep in a pool of tears,
I hear the faint beat of my lonely heart,

> slip-sliding away...
> slip-sliding away.

The Edge Of The World

The music shakes, spills,
falls off the edge of the world
in muted tones and keys.

Moments slow, stop,
collapse
into the eternal now.
Time ceases to exist.

> *Inside this vacuum:*
> *Silence within.*
> *Silence without.*

In this still small space,
I move as wet hard mist
splashing, splintering, scattering
above myself,
below myself,
and yet, within myself.

I peer through
a surreal foggy lens
at nondescript ghosts
moving their lips
in deafening silence.

I perceive a whisper of wings,
a flutter of heartbeats.

> *Inside this vacuum:*
> *Silence within.*
> *Silence without.*

I fall off the edge of the world
in muted tones and keys
into a silence of echoes.

The Fog

With Silent footfalls
I wander these midnight streets,
a ghostly gray figure
blending into the fog.

I become invisible
inside night's hazy envelope.

I drift aimlessly
through the atmosphere's
thick weightless element.

Voices without faces ebb and flow
in a distant tide of unseen strangers.

A siren approaches.
Its desolate scream
      invades,
      passes,
      fades,
swallowed up by the fog.

A creeping damp
chills my ankles,
climbs to my eyes,
makes them wet...

I'm not crying!
I'm not!!

With silent footfalls
I continue walking through midnight,
a ghostly figure
hazing in and out,
slowly, slowly
becoming...
the fog.

The Sands Of Eternity

Caught in the obtuse angle
of a one-sided thought,
my mind circles
in square root patterns
on a canvas of shifting sands.

Sparkles,
sewn into the pale gray carpet I lay on,
form diagonal paths
across the ink-stained pages
of my consciousness.

In the distance,
growing louder as it approaches,
a disembodied flute plays
in a harmony of circular echoes
held in invisible dance,
nuzzling the rain,
blowing kisses onto the wind,
beckoning me to follow.

I walk through sun shadows,
mind strum rainbow songs,
sparkle for a brief moment,
then melt into the sands of eternity.

The Silence

I walk between two golden deer,
flanked by albino wolves,
inside the oneness of our breath.
Ravens and doves circle above,
living auras adorning our souls.

    Beneath a sky of burnished gold,
        beside a lake of diamond dust,
    I stand in awe of heaven's voice.
        Angels and cherubs circle above
misty pharaohs from centuries past.

    I hear the voice of God
        calling to me from the other side
            inside the breath of death.
        A flurry of wings circles above
and a hush falls over the silence.

    I am a lonely dream drifting
through the space time continuum
        inside an ever-changing dimension
        hazing in circles above
the silence between pulse beats.

I move between the here and there,
        flanked by a ring of wandering ghosts
inside this never-ending dream,
        sleepwalking in circles above
           the silence
        between breath and death.

Unsearchable

As the rain falls,
sky tears mingle with mine.
I become one
with this coldest night of nights.

This chill is too encompassing.
This rain is too hard.

Sometimes I feel I'm part of the rain,
or it's a child of mine,
stillborn inside a veil of sorrow.

I'll wrap this rain around me
until I am the rain.

I'll fall softly through oblivion
until I become unsearchable.

Voices

My voice
is a chorus of rattling bones,
taut nerves
and distant dreams.

Liquid...
like slow moving water
over slick black rocks,
beneath timeless bridges,
pressing stone after pebble after stone
against my consciousness.

I am a shadow, a flicker,
interference patterns and sound waves
imprinted on the skin of infinity.

Thirsty for spirit, stars and knowledge
        I dive into the deep,
Ready for that stranger, death,
        to embrace me,
      and crush my voice
through the dark heart of his lament
      until we are both one voice
      and my bones rattle no more.

Oblique

There is a location called mine,
Known, yet unknown to me,
in this place I am,
in this place I will never be.

I am a being,
with no substance or essence,
that is not a being:

        seen but obscure,
        flashing off and on,
        walking with millions
        yet walking alone always.

More here and less there.
More there and less here.
        Entwined in my karma
        far from my destiny.
        All my letters arriving
        in sealed vacuums.

The horizon colours the sky
and colonizes the stars
in glorious surreal architecture.
but in this location of mine,
known yet unknown to me,
I am but will never be.

This is the place of oblique lenses
distorted mirrors and closed doors left ajar,
where it is not possible to enter or exit.

I am here but can never arrive.

        So, it is and will never be.
        So, I am and will ever be
        disposition dislocated
        in lockstep with futility.

Somebody Else's Dream

Running down a quarter line
spinning on a dime,
spending time like water
on a slice of dark sand,
the edges of this circle
are jagged razor blades:
      No beginning.
      No end.

Stuck in the middle,
a hand me down child
wearing thin tears,
is clothed in another's dream.
Not real to the touch.
Constantly phasing and hazing
in foggy burnt embers.

When nobody remembers
your face
or your name.
you just keep running
down that quarter line
hazing in and out
of somebody else's dream,
never your own ...

never your own.

Inversion

Somewhere,
under my shadow,
beneath my feet,
a silent moving sea,
a hidden red volcano,
an invisible reflection
of a parallel mind.

The gift-wrapped Earth
is cautiously hiding
the secret revelations
of an inverted universe ...
somewhere,
under my shadow,
beneath my feet.

In the Valley of Blurred Mirrors

Hiding inside pearls of hard moonlight,
buried deep in a valley of blurred mirrors,
I survive on second hand breath,
holding hands with death
in this shadowy land of haze.

I've outgrown the skin I'm trapped in.
The world turns inside out.
Shapeshifting through the eye of a tear
I emerge in contrasts of myself.

Gray world turned black.
Eclipse of the eyes
lidding open to a distant monolith
slowly approaching,
mirroring
pearls of hard moonlight and death,
wrapped in second hand breath
deep in the valley of blurred mirrors.

... And I am there.

Smoky Dream

Standing inside my shadow,
I peer out into a world that doesn't see me.
Cloaked in my many masks,
I've lost myself too.

Disguised as a ghostly dream,
I am disappearing smoke.
Exhaled, inhaled.
Part of them yet separate
in my ghostly guise.

This shadow land I wander in
is ragged at the edges,
sore to the touch
and cold as ice.

I cling to my masks
and my loneliness
inside this world of shadows.
Nobody can reach me.

I am the smoky dream
thinning at the edges
dissolving into the atmosphere ...
soon to be forever lost to the world.

Face in the Mirror

The face in the mirror
streaked with steam,
is peeking through
the fragments of my visible self
at my invisible self
and the ghost behind me.

Eyes blink
to remove the ghost
that will not disappear.

Hazy face,
familiar eyes
beckon me into the swirl,
into the fantasy crack in the glass,
the crack in my world
that haphazardly intersects
the highway of another dimension.

Choices:
Dimensionalize, disappear,
or blink back into existence.

Lids flutter.
The atmosphere cools.
The mist lifts.
The ghost undresses, disappears.
The mirror gasps, unstreaks.
The last droplet of water evaporates.

I reflect, refract.
unstreak, evaporate
and dissolve ...
into my invisible self
on the other side of the mirror.

Remembering the Rain

I remember the rain:
The texture of its touch.
And the timbre of its voice.

The rain speaks in soft staccato
to the evergreens,
it whispers to the gleaming
graffiti-carved park benches.

An overcast, slow-moving Canadian sky
chases fading clouds across a graying expanse,
and somewhere there is a distant beach
trying to catch up with a summer too far away.

Here, the rain speaks
in many languages and tongues:
In a loud, raspy voice to some.
In soft, gentle whispers to others.

And then it stops
but its lips keep on moving.

Mine stop
and move no more.

When I am dead
remember me ...
remembering the rain.

The Only Moment

(ekphrastic poem written to Angels (Paradise), 1909.
artwork by M.K.Ciurlionis 1875-1910)

A broken winged lament
      has brought me to this moment,
      felled me to my soiled knees.

      I am alone in a throng of spirits,
         surrounded by songs
            and sweet memories.

I cannot lift my head.
      I can only stare at the scattered pebbles,
         disguised as heavenly flowers.

I can feel there is a golden tide of dreams
      just beyond my reach.
I can hear a flutter of wings above me
      just beyond my sight.

      And just behind the shapeshifting clouds,
         I know eternity rests
     in the technicolour palm
of the creator's right hand.

With his left hand,
I can feel him lift his brush of many colours
      breathing life into death
         just beyond this realm.

In my mind
I can see him lifting my head
      and painting me into paradise
         just beyond this moment
           into
        the only moment
        that ever will matter.

The Dream Fulfilled

There's a shrine I visit in my mind.
When I'm lonely I go there to find
those who've passed on and left me alone
but still reside in my twilight zone.

Now day are short and nights are long.
I sleep inside an old lost song.
As time moves slow, I creep along
this path to home where I belong.

There's a special magic in the air
that fills my soul as I enter there.
I see past loves and family;
those who are so dear to me.

My breath's abating by and by.
The dream fulfilled; on wings I'll fly.
Wrapped inside a whisper and sigh,
I'll touch them in the blink of an eye.

The End?

Death

Death is an adult agony.
A burning off of the body
to leave the soul behind.

The coming apart
of Siamese twins.
A painful release at best.

The final breath:
A gasping eventide song
sung with uncertainty.

Death,
our final freedom,
crossed more frighteningly
than thin cracking ice.

Within Me

An angel shot silk
into the heart of the stars
and a universe was born.

The force behind the stone,
the blood within the bone
was the power of God,
creator of the all.

He molds all life
and I am in his keep.

Upon my death,
        I will not die.

Inhale, Exhale

Waving goodbye to it all
there are urchins from my past
squealing with delight as I depart,
and there are tear filled ghosts
lamenting my leaving.

> *Inhale, exhale*
> and keep the weeping
> hushed, hidden and minimal.

I drift aimlessly on the hum of a song
vibrating softly on someone else`s lips.
The tune is familiar yet forgotten.
I can`t quite put a name or a place to the memory.

There comes a distant whisper
too muffled to be deciphered
or channelled into language,
too rare to be bought or sold or understood.
I know it`s meant for me,

> *Inhale, exhale.*
> *Inhale, exhale.*

At the edge of the horizon I see a hazy figure,
    reminiscent of myself; fading fast
    into the slow-motion sunset cascade.

I pass through rivers, sundowns,
    nights and stars,
until I pass through myself

> *Inhale, exhale*
> one last time, this side of heaven,
>   as I wave goodbye to it all.

The Waters of Time

The salt from the ocean
     nips at my eyes
         clawing at yesterday's memories
    scratching my spirit alive.

    I walk the waters of my soul
        on the shorelines of eternity
    adrift in a million reflections
        that warm and chill my heart.

The sun is a dying flamingo
    crashing into the distant horizon
and I am slowly coming alive
    inside thiss dream I have died in.

I move deeper into the waters of time
    to rock in the arms of the ocean
        and rest in the arms of the angels
that have always been calling me home.

As I Lie Underneath and Deep Within

A sudden frost-bound wind
          swirls softly
     through ice-riddled fields of dearth,
       and whistles
        through the whispering pines,
          as I lie underneath
       and deep within.

    The branches snap their fingers
        in stony-faced repose
   to the trance-like rhythm
      of the atmosphere.

The bridge that overlooks the eddying stream
     creaks to the drumbeat
        of a thousand sighs.

I take no heed of brackish gathering clouds
that threaten high above my cold tombstone:
     deaf to all the words you never said,
     dead to all the deeds I left undone,
       as I lie underneath
         and deep within.

The End

I sit on the edge of an hour
     counting the minutes and seconds,
unzipping them into years,
     marking the months and days.

     The days are growing short
and my breath is stretching thin.

I balance on the snowy edge of my thoughts
     and call out to the pale blue tree
that sways against my ice-pocked heart;
     but there is nothing to hold onto,
          not even a forgotten wish.

     As I fade into the Netherlands
          of death's cruel surprise,
             the last thing I feel
        is winter's chilled breath
     scratching at the door of my heart;
        its echo cracking the dream
and my soul
        fading, fading
          just ...
             fading away.

A Cold Crisp Morning

Walking the beach on a cold crisp morning
a damp sky above imposes a warning.
Storm clouds droop in pale shades of gray
as a wild wind threatens to blow them away.

There's a bittersweet taste in mouth and dreams.
A sugary acid that tears at their seams.
I can feel the chill of second-hand breath
in this season of winter's impending death.

So, I walk a bit faster, try to outrun the rain
even though every step is riddled with pain.
These old knees have walked too many roads
and my back is aching from too many loads.

I hear a gull's lamentable cry.
I see an eagle soaring on high.
As a beautiful feather falls from the sky
a sorrowful teardrop falls from my eye
for the sun-swept beaches of yesterday
and the glory days that have faded away

I've been waiting for what dreams may come.
Wishing on falling stars, coming undone.

And now too much time has come and gone.
These old eyes won't witness another dawn.
So, I throw off my coat on this cold crisp morning
and pay no attention to the sky's dark warning.

Age's caught me off-guard and handcuffed my wrists.
My body's dissolving in teardrops and mists.
Storm clouds rip open and drown the day
and the wild wind of death blows me away.

The wild wind of death ... just blows me away.

The Corner of Dark and Night

A dozen helium balloons
glide over the glistening bay,
above the sails and pontoons
that bob and slap and sway.

Red, and yellow, green and white.
They hold my eyes fast, hypnotized.
The sun relinquishes its light
imprisoned in twilight's demise.

The day falls into night's embrace,
succumbs to dark, loses its light.
In shame day hides her guilty face
inside the charcoal chest of the night.

Each twinkling star's a stepping stone.
Each thought a word. Each word a poem.
A silent song inside a prayer.
An angels' choir is leading me there.

Inside this dark I'm not alone.
I'm past twilight. I'm coming home.
I turn the corner of dark and night,
and finally walk into the light.

Door of the Dead

On this stretch of deserted beach
the sand is gleaming and singing
      songs to the sun and the sea.

I am as quiet as pooled water:
restless without wind,
      listless without movement.

I float through the haze of my non-existent days,
a slick liquid satin on the waters of life
      reflecting the rainfall of days past.

At the light violet edge of approaching twilight
I encroach on the tender lip of the night;
        a shadow in a shadow,
      casting a shadow
onto the fading sun.

On this stretch of deserted beach
I am gleaming and singing songs
     to the sun
        and the sea
           ... and the dead.

I lift up my eyes
     to the stars overhead
         and enter the door of the dead.

Amber Glow and White Light

In the dim of the sanctuary at midnight
the amber glow split into pristine white light.
In a rhythmic twist it moved into sound.
With a subconscious motion it scattered around.
The elegant air was singing in tune
at the star dusted edge of a November moon.
And I knew it was time for my prayer to be heard
so, I uttered it loud without saying a word.

It was then I saw you swaying down low
with eloquent words in the sweet amber glow.
In this surreal moment of bittersweet pain
I felt the warm nuzzle of yesterday's rain.
And my cup overflowed with mercy and love.
A sacrament from the Great Realm above.

The sky was aglow with papers and dust
and memories alive with old songs and rust.
The mouth of the universe opened up wide
and begged me enter on its rising tide.
I took off my lifejacket, threw it away.
I buried my ego and my feet of clay.

In the dim sanctuary just past midnight
the amber glow split into pristine white light.
I entered heaven in the blink of an eye
And oh, oh ... what a beautiful sight ...
　　　　oh, what a beautiful sight.

Inn of the Seventh Tranquility

And now...
the final journey begins.
I walk through powdered rose petals
on a stretch of silver sand,
travelling with ghosts from my past
and familiar angels,
to the Inn of The Seventh Tranquility.

Under a metallic translucent sky
the coo of a snow-white dove
drifts on the whisper of the waves.
Beneath a forgiving sun,
I see the gold dusted pathway
leading to the Inn of The Seventh Tranquility

I can see clearly now.
Through the years of indecision,
the moments of indiscretion,
faulty choices and wasted days and nights
my compass point has remained magnetized
drawing me unwittingly
yet relentlessly, to my destiny.

Through the heartaches and tears,
laughter and smiles, successes and failures
from the depths of despair to the heights of success
coming full circle and repeating again.
the unchangeable karma and wheels of precision
carry me to the Inn of the Seventh Tranquility.

At the last steps, weary and fragile,
I am lifted from the veiled mists of life
by a flurry of wings
to the Inn of the Seventh Tranquility
where I rest in the arms of the angels
as the final journey ends.

Liquid Flame

A passionate moment in time
passes through itself,
collapses into my soul.
A sweet taste
whets my lips
as rain falls,
shines the day
to a fine gloss.

A straw tinder box of abstractions
kindles itself into glorious flame,
anointing my feet
that I may keep pace
with a new quickening
that burns in an orchestration
of deafening silences.

Inside the surreal breath
of this invisible rhythm
I embrace the ringing in my ears
and dance through a magical weave
of sparkling water and wine
in a strange familiar ceremony
of forgotten dreams
spinning real.

In the wake of distant thunder
the tinder box turns to ash.

An angel's wing grazes my soul.
The angel whispers my name.

I turn to liquid flame.

Justified Water

Cleanse me in justified water.
Let ice cold needles puncture my heart
that i may die to myself,
then, resurrect me to walk again
in the brightest corner of light
where shadows flee and hide
from the truth chasing them down,
then send in the angels
to lighten my load
and clear the pathway ahead.

Let me stand justified
on the water you lay down before me.
Breathe your essence into me
that I may be you.
and see myself through your eyes.

As I slowly sink into the justified water,
the water you lay down before me,
the last thing I see
is my waiting spirit
as I melt into its essence
and gently embrace the drowning.

Night's Beaujolais Wine

In the heartland glitter of sage and shine
night falls like dark red Beaujolais wine.
Hiding the beauty and scent of the rose
the sky's eyes flutter then slowly close.

Beneath the sudden descent of darkness,
clouds fall to their knees and start to undress.
A sacred vibration awakens the sky
as throngs of angels slowly pass by.

Then the night's dark Beaujolais wine ebbs away
into the dawn of a sage and shine day.
The dew on the rose fades then disappears
as the sun reaches down to dry her tears.

Hazing above the horizon line
I flow in the wake of a smooth white wine.
Swinging new songs, I sway with the old
'til the heat of the music abates and grows cold.

Life on a string, spun then unspun,
the day's growing weary and coming undone.
I've had my glory my time in the sun
I've passed the baton; my race has been run.

So long I've sojourned in life's lost and found.
Now, moving through lights, music and sound
I stand in the quick of night's Beaujolais wine
in awe of God's grandeur and noble design.

After I've Gone

I will be gone when you wake tomorrow,
But I do not leave you empty hearted.

To you my love, I leave:

My thoughts to mingle with your daydreams
that you may resist the reality that I have really gone.
My words to echo in your castigated ears
that grew conveniently deaf as I spoke of my truths.
My stone-cold silence to your icy lips
that have so casually bruised my heart.
My second sight to your fragile artistic fingers
that they may try to paint the love I offered you.
And, finally, my four bank accounts with nothing in them
that you may empty them when you're in need.

And:

I leave my misdirected passion
To the broken-hearted and down-trodden spirits,
Still searching for a Nirvana that cannot be found,

To the ragamuffins and beggars in the street,
living in back alleys alive with a million lacklustre eyes,
I leave wishes owed to me that I failed to collect.

To my fair-weather friends, paper kings
and cut-out doll queens,
I leave the meaningless ambitions and fleeting fame
I found lying beside a graffiti-scarred dumpster,

To everyone:

I will be gone when you wake tomorrow,
but I do not leave empty hearted.
        No, I do not leave empty hearted.
            I was ... a poet!

AFTERTHOUGHT

The Cane

A multi-coloured sparkling cane
stands beside the open door.
Will it ever walk again?
Or stand alone forevermore.

If only that bright cane could talk.
Would it speak of better days?
When they went on their morning walk?
When she was not lost in a haze?

The cane would ask, "Where has she gone?"
in tones despairing and bereft.
"I don't hear her familiar song
and I'm so lonely since she left."

The universe would hear her cry
and gently touch her handle grip;
and whisper in a tender sigh
with a slightly trembling lip,

"She's gone to heaven high above
and won't be coming back again.
She's wrapped inside God's tender love.
She's happy now and has no pain."

And if that sparkling cane could speak,
it would say "God bless her soul."
A tear would grace its shiny cheek ...
Nevermore would they stroll.

AFTERWORD

Higher

I've walked the summer pathways
of love when it's in bloom
And travelled down its alleys
of heartaches, tears and gloom.
I've walked through dreams with passion
pulling at my sleeve
And learned that love is all that matters.
This is my belief.

I've held a baby in my arms
and been blessed by its breath.
I've come to trust the Lord
and have no of fear death.
I've climbed inside compassion
that fit me like a glove.
I've given up my heart and soul
for the sake of love.

I've had my share of heartaches
but faith has seen me through
The darkest of the starkest nights
into a sky of blue.
It's been a destined journey,
a long walk to remember
Under summer sunsets,
through snowstorms in December.

> *And now the days are hazing grey,*
> *shorter every one.*
> *Winter's chill is gaining ground.*
> *The sun is on the run...*

Looking back upon my life
I do have some regrets
but I never hedged my bets.
and always paid my debts
The teardrops falling down my cheek
reflect each smile and frown.
The final days are drawing near.
The sun is going down.

I've tried to run the good race
and when my life is done
I hope my words will still find life
on someone else's tongue
And if perchance they soothe a heart
or cause a lover's sigh,
Higher on an angel's wing
this soul of mine will fly.

AUTHOR PROFILE

Candice James is a poet, visual artist, singer/songwriter, musician, workshop facilitator and book reviewer for Canadian Poetry Review and Pacific Rim Review of Books. She completed her 2nd three year term as Poet Laureate of The City of New Westminster, BC CANADA in June 2016 and was appointed Poet Laureate Emerita in November 2016 by order of City Council. She is Founder of: Royal City Literary Arts Society; Fred Cogswell Award for Excellence in Poetry; Poetry In The Park; Poetry New Westminster; Poetic Justice, and Slam Central. She is Past President of the Federation of British Columbia Writers; Past Director of SpoCan and a full member of the League of Canadian Poets. Candice has judged the "Pat Lowther Memorial Award"; "Jessamy Stursberg -Youth Poet Award" and "Fred Cogswell Award for Excellence in Poetry. She received Pandora's Collective Citizenship Award and Chamber of Commerce Platinum award: the Bernie Legge Artist/Cultural award.

Her poetry has been translated into Arabic, Italian, Bengali, Chinese and Farsi. Her artwork has appeared in Duende Magazine and in Spotlight" Goddard College of Fine Arts, Vermont, USA; her poetry and artwork ("Unmasked") in Survision Magazine, Dublin, Ireland also in Wax Poetry Art Magazine Canada and CQ Magazine USA.

WEBSITE www.candicejames.com
YouTube
https://www.youtube.com/channel/UC2EA5GcEClGYuF3o2K KHJFQ
FACEBOOK Poet Laureate Emerita Page
https://www.facebook.com/NWPoLoEmerita
FACEBOOK Artist Page
https://www.facebook.com/CandiceJamesArtist
FACEBOOK Musician Page
https://www.facebook.com/Candice-James-Songwriter-Bass-Guitarist156859754352277
Twitter:
@NWPoLoEmerita and   @candice23809987

NEIGHBOURS:
THREE SOCIAL SETTLEMENTS
IN DOWNTOWN TORONTO

Allan Irving, Harriet Parsons
and Donald Bellamy

Canadian Scholars' Press Inc.   Toronto   1995

Neighbours: Three Social Settlements in Downtown Toronto

First published in 1995 by
Canadian Scholars' Press Inc.
180 Bloor St. W., Ste. 402,
Toronto, Ontario   M5S 2V6

Canadian Cataloguing in Publication Data

Irving, Allan
      Neighbours: three social settlements in downtown Toronto

Includes bibliographical references and index.
ISBN 1-55130-049-4

1. Social settlements – Ontario – Toronto – History.
2. Social service – Ontario – Toronto – History.
I. Parsons, Harriet. II. Bellamy, Donald F.,
1927–   . III. Title.

HV4200.T617   1995   361.9713'541   C95-930205–0

Cover photograph courtesy of Central Neighbourhood House

Page layout and cover design by Brad Horning

Printed and bound in Canada